Diabetic Cookbook
for Two

QUICK START GUIDE

Whether you're new to managing diabetes for yourself or a family member, or are just looking for some new recipes to incorporate into your existing health management regimen, *Diabetic Cookbook for Two* can help with great tips, ideas, and recipes. Following are five key reasons you'll be glad you read on:

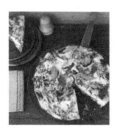

Simplify your life.

Managing diabetes can feel overwhelming, and the time spent in self-care—checking blood sugar, taking medications, being active, and deciding what to eat—can feel like a part-time job! This cookbook will help simplify your life and make managing your diabetes easier with its wholesome recipes perfectly portioned for two people. Gone is the guesswork when cooking for two—your dishes will turn out just right and you'll enjoy eating what's good for you.

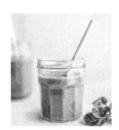

Easy and delicious low-carbohydrate recipes.

Each recipe fits into a low-carb diabetic meal plan and includes a complete nutritional analysis. The recipes have *no more than 45 grams of carbohydrate per serving*. They are also low in total fat, saturated fat, and cholesterol, and high in vitamins, minerals, and fiber, with an emphasis on complex carbohydrates and lean proteins.

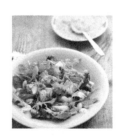

Ban the bland and enjoy your classic favorites revamped.

Having diabetes doesn't mean you have to eat bland food or give up your favorite dishes. Find comfort classics like Mock Mac and Cheese (page 88), Eggplant Lasagna (page 93), and Lazy Turkey Potpie (page 98), redone to be diabetic friendly, portioned for two, and bursting with flavor.

No-stress-added, easy-to-make recipes.

Eating healthy doesn't have to be difficult or time consuming, and you won't need to go to cooking school to become a chef. The recipes in this book are easy to make and contain commonly available ingredients.

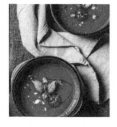

Useful information.

Each recipe contains descriptors with helpful tips, ingredient variations, and serving suggestions. You will learn something with each recipe that can help you become more knowledgeable about the nutrients in the foods you eat. You can then make healthier food decisions at home and in other situations such as eating out or when enjoying family favorites.

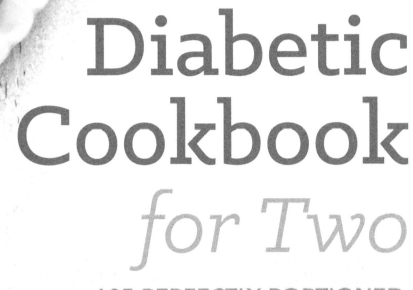

Diabetic Cookbook
for Two

125 PERFECTLY PORTIONED, HEART HEALTHY, LOW-CARB RECIPES

ROCKRIDGE
PRESS

Jennifer Koslo, RD

For general information on our other products and services or to obtain technical support, please contact our Customer Care Department within the U.S. at (866) 744-2665, or outside the U.S. at (510) 253-0500.

Rockridge Press publishes its books in a variety of electronic and print formats. Some content that appears in print may not be available in electronic books, and vice versa.

TRADEMARKS: Rockridge Press and the Rockridge Press logo are trademarks or registered trademarks of Callisto Media Inc. and/or its affiliates, in the United States and other countries, and may not be used without written permission. All other trademarks are the property of their respective owners. Rockridge Press is not associated with any product or vendor mentioned in this book.

Interior photo credits: Victoria Firmston/StockFood, pg. 2, 46; Darren Muir/Stocksy, pg. 2, 66; Gräfe & Unzer Verlag and Anke Schütz/StockFood, pg. 2, 104; Beatrice Peltre/StockFood, pg. 3; Emoke Szabo/Stocksy, pg. 7; Jill Chen/Shutterstock, pg. 8; Successo Images/Shutterstock, pg. 13; Stacey Newman/Shutterstock, pg. 13; Hongchanstudio/Shutterstock, pg. 13; Lumina/Stocksy, pg. 18; Jim Scherer/StockFood, pg. 86; Teleginatania/Shutterstock, pg. 130; Eising Studio/StockFood, pg. 152; Alicia Mañas Aldaya/StockFood, pg. 174; Valerie Janssen/StockFood, pg. 198.

Cover photo credits: Front Cover: People Pictures/StockFood; back cover: Darren Muir/Stocksy, Gräfe & Unzer Verlag and Anke Schütz/StockFood, Victoria Firmston/StockFood.

Print ISBN: 978-1-62315-607-7 | eBook ISBN: 978-1-62315-608-4

CONTENTS

INTRODUCTION

I f you or a loved one has been diagnosed recently with diabetes, you may be struggling with what to cook and how to eat. You may also find it difficult to reconcile "living to eat" versus "eating to live." In the past, diabetic diets were restrictive and complicated. Times, however, have changed. It's likely you'll have to make changes to the foods you eat and portion sizes. You can still eat your favorite foods, however, with a little preparation and planning. *Diabetic Cookbook for Two* is for type 1 and type 2 diabetics who want to prepare simple, healthy meals without using complicated tools.

Eating to manage diabetes means eating a variety of nutritious foods, including vegetables, fruits, nonfat dairy products, whole grains, healthy fats, beans, and lean meats. Moderation is key in both the types of foods you eat and the amounts, as is regularly spacing meals throughout the day—and not skipping meals.

This cookbook contains *125 easy-to-prepare recipes* that are low in fat and carbohydrates without the use of sugars, yet packed with nutrition and bursting with flavor. The recipes do the work of modifying less nutritious recipes designed for a crowd to be perfectly portioned for two—with no waste or unnecessary expenses.

Chapter 1 begins with tips on sharing cooking responsibilities so you spend less time in the kitchen and more time enjoying good-tasting foods and activities. You will learn to create meal plans. Becoming skilled at cooking a new way can be tough. Having a plan can help. Tips for grocery shopping and stocking a diabetic-friendly kitchen are also covered so you can apply what you learn and create meals in a snap.

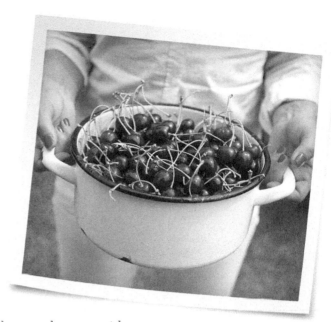

Chapter 2 covers the basics of managing diabetes through diet. You'll learn the connection between the foods you eat and your health. Learning to pick foods rich in vitamins, minerals, and fiber over processed foods can reduce your risk for complications, such as stroke and heart disease. A good diabetes meal plan should be both flexible and practical.

You will need to monitor your daily intake of carbohydrates, though. The pros and cons of different carbohydrate-tracking techniques are discussed. Each recipe's nutritional analysis helps you see how it fits into your overall meal plan. You'll also find tips on everything including grocery shopping, healthier cooking techniques, and incorporating regular physical activity into your life.

Read on to discover healthy and delicious diabetic recipes designed just for two. There are recipes for breakfast, meal-size salads, soups and stews, comfort classics, vegetarian entrées, chicken and fish dishes, pork and beef dinners, and sides and staples. You'll feel so much better when you take control of your blood sugar and manage your diabetes and health.

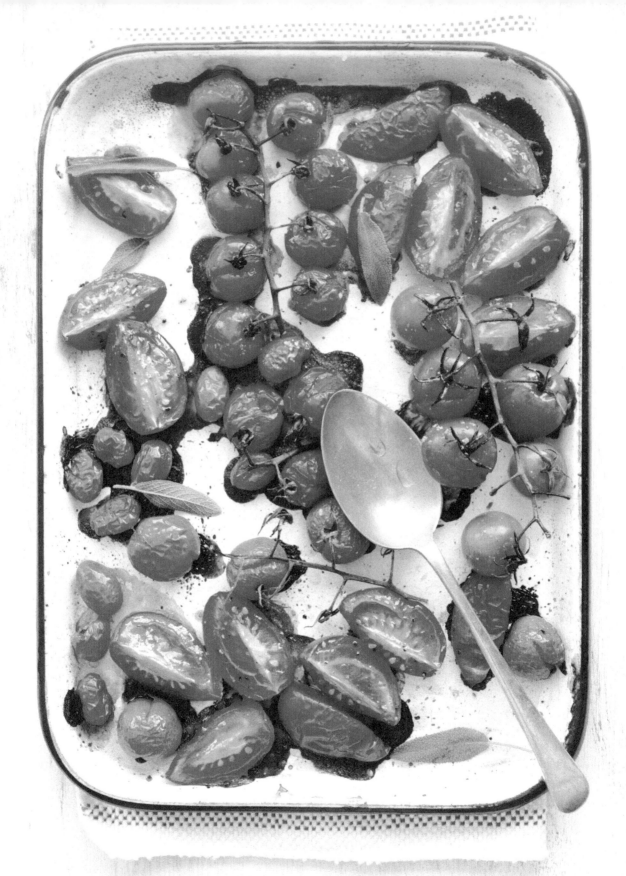

CHAPTER 1

Cooking for Two

Cooking Is Caring

Being diagnosed with type 1 or type 2 diabetes changes your life and can be very scary at times. It certainly isn't the end, however, and you are not alone. There is a lot to learn about managing your blood glucose, taking medications, and how the foods you eat affect your blood-glucose levels. By educating yourself to prepare nutritious wholesome foods and learning a few key skills, you will be well prepared to handle this new way of life.

The good news is that cooking for someone with diabetes, whether yourself or someone else, is really just a commitment to healthy cooking on a day-to-day basis. *A diabetes diet is simply a healthy eating plan high in nutrients, low in fat, and moderate in calories.* The only difference is you need to pay more attention to your food choices—most notably carbohydrates.

Change is hard, but it's never too late to have a positive effect on your diabetes. The important thing to remember is that you *do* have control over your health. And, you can still enjoy your favorite foods and take pleasure from meals without feeling deprived. Learning new skills will help you reestablish a sense of control over your life. It is important to remain optimistic. Look at your health challenge as an opportunity for growth and improving your health, as well as the well-being of others in your household.

Embrace the journey ahead. It will teach you about the nutritional content of foods, the importance of reading labels, and how to cook foods to maintain nutrient content while limiting excess saturated fat, sodium, and empty calories.

Lastly, enlist support and work with your spouse or loved one through this challenge. In addition to learning new skills, it's really an opportunity to grow together. To help you start your journey on the right foot, here are 10 ways to divvy up cooking for the week.

Ten Ways to Divide the Labor of Cooking

When cooking for more than just yourself, the tasks become easier if you share the responsibilities. Consider these suggestions:

1 **Create a list.** Sit down with your loved one and brainstorm a list of tasks you need to do each week to plan, shop, prep, and cook a week's worth of meals. Remember to include the little things, too, like checking expiration dates on those jars in the very back of the refrigerator and checking your freezer for any "mystery" items.

2 **Task timing.** Once you have all the tasks listed, outline the expected frequency as well as the standards expected. For example, one person may think that dishes need to be done at the end of the day while the other thinks once a week is fine.

3 **Plan it and post it.** One of your tasks should be to set aside time each week to decide on a menu and create a shopping list after doing a pantry review. Place a small whiteboard in the kitchen and post the menu so everyone knows the plan for the week. Check your local grocery store sale flyer and make time to pick up items you need.

4 **Cater to talents and embrace specialization.** Instead of dividing chores along stereotypical lines, give the responsibility to the person who is most passionate about the task. Decide who does what job well. Maybe your spouse is better at picking out fresh vegetables or is just a faster shopper overall.

5 **Rotate the jobs neither of you enjoys.** Cleaning out the pantry or taking out the garbage may not be something you are passionate about, but it is necessary. Take turns on those jobs that no one wants to do all the time.

6 **Pick a day to cook together.** Being committed to eating healthy, nutritious foods on a daily basis can help you manage your diabetes. Pick a day when you don't have to work or have fewer obligations and spend a few hours in the kitchen with your spouse learning new recipes and preparing for the week ahead.

7   **Encourage the effort or embrace the task!** A key to avoiding conflict in the kitchen (and beyond!) is to give each person the authority to do assigned tasks in his or her way. If you feel the need to redo the other's task, then the division of chores may need to be redone.

8   **Give your partner a break.** Many couples aim for a 50-50 split of chores, but there's no hard and fast way to keep things "fair." The goal is for each person involved to feel supported by the other. There are days when diabetes affects mood and energy level. Instead of feeling resentful, give your partner a break. Nothing says I love you like, "I'll do that for you today."

9   **Verbalize appreciation and keep a sense of humor.** Remember to go with the flow and keep a sense of humor. If the breakfast oatmeal is a little burned, and the dinner chicken is a little dry, laugh, take it in stride, and use it as an opportunity to build memories together.

10 **Enlist help.** Finally, if you need help, consider asking your children, siblings, neighbors, or friends. Check with your local diabetes association to see if there are families interested in doing a meal swap or supper club where you team up with other families so you only have to cook once or twice a week.

How to Plan for a Week

When cooking for two, heating a microwave dinner or grabbing takeout sounds much easier than whipping up a home-cooked meal. Years of spontaneous food choices may make the idea of planning meals for a week seem a bit tedious and unappealing. There are definitely advantages, though—particularly in terms of decreasing your risk for health complications. Cooking healthy meals at home can help you control your diabetes and your weight. It really is amazing what health-conscious eating, combined with physical activity, can do for preventing the progression of this disease. Think of a meal plan as a road map to healthy eating and living.

Planning meals in advance and knowing what you'll eat for breakfast, lunch, and dinner each day make it far less likely that you'll get off track with your diet. With easy and delicious recipes, making meals from scratch ensures you are eating wholesome food. You control the ingredients so you know exactly what's in each meal. In addition to being easy to prepare, the recipes in this book each contain a nutritional breakdown so you can easily see how each meal fits with your individualized meal plan.

Meal planning saves money, too! By shopping from a list, you are less likely to make those impulse purchases and you'll be done shopping sooner. You'll also save money because you will waste less food. Most people throw away a lot of food from their weekly shopping trips. You can avoid this with meal planning. Anything left over from one meal can be eaten for lunch or as a snack the next day.

Most of us have food lingering in our cupboards that is perfectly edible but hasn't been used for one reason or another. You won't have to worry about adding to that stash when you use the recipes in this book. If a recipe calls for an ingredient that will yield an unused portion, the recipe includes a "Toss it Together Tip" so you can incorporate purchased items into other meals.

With a little organization and effort, meal planning can slow the progression of diabetes, help your family eat healthier, and save you time and money! Let's get started with meal planning. Following is an example of dinners for two for one week.

SAMPLE WEEKLY MEAL PLAN: DINNER

DAY	MEAL
Monday	Chickpea-Spinach Curry
Tuesday	Meatloaf for Two
Wednesday	Freshened-Up French Onion Soup
Thursday	Gingered-Pork Stir-Fry
Friday	Fish Tacos
Saturday	Peppered Beef with Greens and Beans
Sunday	Portobello Mushroom Pizzas

SHOPPING LIST FOR SAMPLE WEEKLY MEAL PLAN

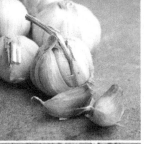

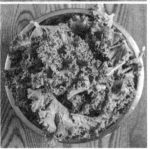

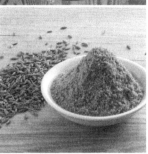

DAIRY AND EGGS

➤ Eggs

➤ Nonfat milk

➤ Mozzarella cheese, shredded nonfat

➤ Swiss cheese, shredded nonfat

GROCERY

➤ Almond meal

➤ Beef broth, low-sodium

➤ Broccoli florets, frozen

➤ Cashews

➤ Chickpeas, canned

➤ Chinese rice wine

➤ Corn tortillas

➤ Flaxseed, finely ground

➤ Green beans, frozen

➤ Red wine vinegar

➤ Sesame oil

➤ Soy sauce, low-sodium

➤ Spinach, frozen

➤ Stevia, granulated

➤ Tomatoes, canned chopped

➤ Tomato paste

➤ Tomato sauce

➤ Worcestershire sauce

PANTRY ITEMS

➤ Basil, dried

➤ Black pepper, freshly ground

➤ Cayenne pepper

➤ Cumin, ground

➤ Curry powder

➤ Garlic, granulated and cloves

➤ Extra-virgin olive oil

➤ Extra-virgin olive oil cooking spray

➤ Oregano, dried

➤ Red pepper flakes

➤ Sage, dried

➤ Salt

➤ Thyme, dried

PRODUCE

➤ Avocado

➤ Basil, fresh

➤ Bell peppers, various colors

➤ Cilantro, fresh

➤ Ginger, fresh

➤ Kale

➤ Mushrooms, any variety

➤ Olives, black

➤ Onions, yellow and red

➤ Parsley, fresh

➤ Portobello mushroom caps

➤ Snow peas

➤ Tomatoes, large

MEAT

➤ Boneless sirloin

➤ Ground beef

➤ Lean pork

➤ Tilapia

3   **Eggs:** Eggs are a perfect protein for breakfast, lunch, and dinner. Eggs work great in low-carb crêpes and pancakes and can make putting together a quick, healthy meal of frittatas, scrambled eggs, or omelets a snap! For added nutrition, look for eggs fortified with heart-healthy omega-3 fats.

4   **Frozen vegetables and fruits:** Having frozen fruits and vegetables on hand cuts down on prep time and food waste. Thaw only what you need for each recipe. Frozen fruits and vegetables are picked at their prime and have more flavor and nutrients than fresh produce purchased out of season. Even better, there's no added sodium or sugar contained in canned vegetables and fruits.

5   **Ground flaxseed:** Flaxseed is very low in carbohydrates and high in fiber, which makes it an excellent choice for diabetics. This low-carb food is high in heart-healthy omega-3 fats and makes the perfect complement to most meals. Flaxseed can be mixed into breakfast dishes, used in smoothies, sprinkled on salads, used as a breading substitute, and shaken onto steamed vegetables for a nutty flavor.

6   **Plain nonfat Greek yogurt:** Incorporating dairy products in your diet can be a great way to get calcium and high-quality protein. For diabetics, Greek yogurt is an exceptional meal and snack option due to its low-carbohydrate and high-protein content. Greek yogurt is great for breakfast, in smoothies, on low-carb pancakes, and enjoyed as a snack. It can also replace sour cream in dips and recipes due to its similar taste and texture. Opt for nonfat plain varieties to limit added sugars. You can stir in a bit of stevia if you need that extra bit of sweetness.

7   **Nuts:** Nuts are full of heart-healthy fats and make great toppings for breakfast dishes. Or throw them in smoothies, eat as snacks, toss in salads, and even use as a flour substitute for breading. Storing nuts in the freezer is better than storing them in the pantry. It prevents the oils from going rancid. They don't take long to thaw—just set them on the counter for about 10 minutes and they're ready to eat.

8   **Old-fashioned rolled oats:** Old-fashioned oats are a healthy source of complex carbohydrates and are rich in soluble fiber, which is associated with a decreased risk of heart disease. Old-fashioned oats can also help you feel full longer because of their high fiber content. As a result, they are a beneficial part of a weight-loss plan. Oats are considered a low–glycemic index food. Eating a breakfast of old-fashioned oats can help stabilize blood sugar. Oats work well in pancakes and smoothies and as a bread crumb substitute.

9   **Prewashed salad greens:** Keep a bag or two of prewashed mixed greens on hand to give your lunches and dinners a quick nutritional boost. Just add a dash of extra-virgin olive oil and seasonings or enjoy them with nothing at all!

10 **Quinoa** (pronounced *keen-wah*): Quinoa is a great rice substitute, rich in fiber and protein—and gluten-free. It only takes 15 minutes to cook. Buy pre-rinsed quinoa if you can. If not, always rinse the seeds thoroughly in water before cooking to remove its natural bitter coating. Quinoa is a seed eaten like a whole grain. It can be mixed with fruits, nuts, cinnamon, and nondairy milk for breakfast, used as a base for a meal-size salad, or as a high-fiber, high-protein carbohydrate at dinner.

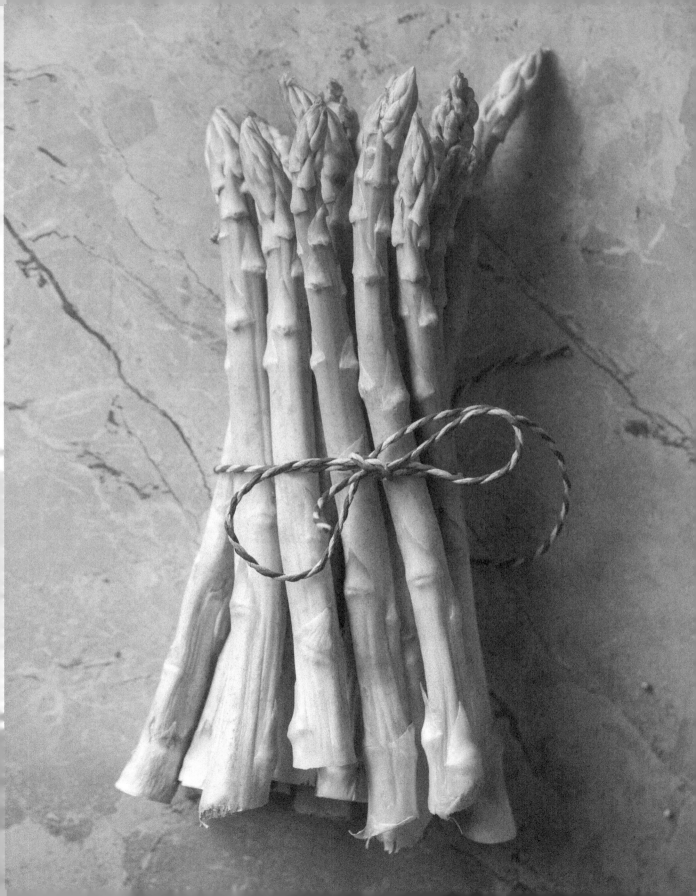

Delicious Diabetic Cooking

CHAPTER 2

You've Been Diagnosed, Now What?

Being diagnosed with diabetes can be confusing and overwhelming. There are many new things to learn and understand. In most cases, your diabetes care team will be there to support you, but the day-to-day management of your diabetes will be in your hands. Topping the list of self-care behaviors you will need to become skilled at are healthy eating and being active.

Healthy eating means consuming foods that provide all three nutrients in reasonable amounts to help you achieve and maintain a healthy body weight. They are:

1. Carbohydrates
2. Fat
3. Protein

It means eating *regularly spaced* meals that are low in saturated fat and sodium. It also means being consistent with the amount and type of carbohydrates you eat at one time.

What it doesn't mean is giving up your favorite foods for nothing but bland boiled vegetables for the rest of your life! Trimming portion sizes, cutting out saturated and trans fats, substituting unsweetened, lower-calorie beverages for soda or sweet tea, and switching out high-sodium processed foods for whole foods may do the trick. But making these changes may require a healthy eating refresher.

Rethinking Your Kitchen Staples

To refresh your diet, you need to know the nutrient content of foods (especially carbohydrates), how to read foods labels, how to stock a healthy pantry, and how to cook foods to maintain their nutrient content while avoiding extra saturated fat and sodium.

To set yourself up for success, focus on the concept of addition rather than subtraction, and adding color, variety, and freshness to your diet. Subtracting foods has such a negative connotation. And, really, your goal is to improve your health by *adding* antioxidant-rich foods so you feel great, have more energy, stabilize your mood, and most importantly, stabilize your blood sugar.

Overhauling your diet overnight isn't realistic and usually leads to frustration and the urge to give up. Instead, start slowly and make simple changes over time, like adding a salad to your diet once a day or switching from butter to extra-virgin olive oil when cooking. Another place to start is your pantry. Donate highly processed prepackaged foods made with white flour, salt, preservatives, and added fats. You don't have to be perfect; the long-term goal is to reduce your risk of cancer and diabetic complications. Every positive change you make to your diet—no matter how small—counts.

Carbs, Sugar, and You

Carbohydrates are one of the three nutrients that make up the foods we eat (fat and protein are the other two). We need carbohydrates to live—they are our primary source of energy and the only fuel source that our brains can use. The problem is there is so much hype about carbohydrates that people get the impression they are bad. Considering carbs is especially confusing for diabetics because eating carbs can mean a rise in blood sugar. But carbs are important, and here are a few things you need to know:

➤   Carbs are found in three basic food groups—sugars, starches, and fiber—and come in two basic forms: simple and complex. Simple carbohydrates are sugars and refined flours, while complex carbohydrates consist of starches and fiber.

➤   Starchy foods like potatoes, rice, and pasta, and sweet foods like sugar and honey, are high in carbohydrates.

➤   Sugar is not the enemy—sugar is just one type of carbohydrate. It's the total carb count that has the most impact on blood-sugar levels. So it's okay to have a small dessert, on occasion; just count it as part of your daily carbohydrate allowance.

➤   The majority of your carb choices should be whole and unprocessed and high in fiber. Fiber is a special form of carbohydrate that you will want to include more of because we don't digest it. Fiber binds to fat and sugar, slowing down absorption, resulting in more even blood-sugar levels.

TYPE 1 VERSUS TYPE 2 DIABETES

HOW ARE THEY DIFFERENT?

Both types of diabetes result from a disruption in the body's natural production and use of insulin, a hormone that moves carbohydrates (sugar) from the blood to the cells. In people with type 1 diabetes (formerly called juvenile-onset or insulin-dependent diabetes), the body does not produce insulin. People with type 2 diabetes have too little insulin, or the body cannot use it effectively.

With type 1 diabetes, the body's immune system destroys the cells that release insulin, eventually eliminating it from the body. Type 1 diabetics take required insulin injections to move sugar out of the bloodstream. This type of diabetes is a result of a virus or autoimmune disorder and cannot be prevented. Symptoms start in childhood and it is usually diagnosed before age 40.

Type 2 diabetes (formerly called adult-onset or non-insulin-dependent diabetes), can develop at any age, but most commonly develops in adulthood. With type 2 diabetes, the cells become resistant to the actions of insulin and the body becomes less efficient at moving sugar out of the bloodstream, resulting in high blood sugar. Type 2 diabetes is associated with obesity and low physical activity. Unfortunately, it is on the rise in children. Type 2 diabetes can be prevented or delayed by living a healthy lifestyle, losing weight and maintaining a healthy weight, following a healthy diet, and exercising regularly.

Both types of diabetes drastically increase a person's risk for serious health complications, including stroke, blindness, kidney failure, heart disease, and foot and leg amputations.

Food Exchanges versus Counting Carbs

Carbohydrates are measured in units called grams. The total grams or amount of carbohydrates you need each day depends on your calorie goals, activity level, and personal preferences. There are several ways people with diabetes can manage food intake to keep blood sugar within their target range, including the food exchange system and carbohydrate counting.

In the food exchange system, food is categorized into three main groups:

1.   Carbohydrates
2.   Protein and protein substitutes
3.   Fats

The **carbohydrate group** is further broken down into bread/starch, fruit, milk, other carbohydrates (sugar and sweets), and vegetables.

Within each food group, foods with similar amounts of carbohydrate per serving size are grouped together. The foods within each group can be "exchanged" for one another during meal planning, giving you about the same amount of carbohydrate.

One carbohydrate exchange (bread/starch, fruit, milk) equals 15 grams of carbohydrate. Since a serving of vegetables has only 5 grams of carbohydrates, it takes 3 vegetables to equal 1 carbohydrate exchange.

For example, if a meal plan says 2½ carbohydrate exchanges, using a food exchange list, you would make your choices. It could look something like: 1 slice of bread, 1 medium peach, and ½ cup of milk. Or you might choose ½ cup of cooked pasta, 1 cup of cubed melon, and ½ cup of nonfat yogurt.

A disadvantage of this method is that it can be difficult to understand and the exchanges may not be exact. As a result, the American Diabetes Association typically recommends carbohydrate counting for managing carbohydrate intake. With carbohydrate counting, you work with your dietitian to plan how many carbohydrates to eat at meals and with snacks. When you know how many grams of carbohydrates you need at each meal, you can choose from any of the three carbohydrate-containing food groups to meet your allowance: bread/starch, fruit, vegetable, and milk. With the carbohydrate counting method, you use the information on food labels to help you select your foods, making this system more accurate, easier, and more flexible.

Each recipe in *Diabetic Cookbook for Two* contains a complete nutritional analysis so you can see how it fits into your day's allowance. The recipes all have a total carbohydrate count of 45 grams or less per serving.

Healthy Cooking Techniques

Healthy cooking doesn't require that you be a trained chef or invest in expensive cookware. In fact, you may already be using many of the techniques that follow. When you prepare and cook meals at home, you have more control over the nutritional content and overall healthiness of the foods you eat. The healthy cooking techniques described here best capture the flavor and retain the nutrients in foods without adding excessive amounts of fats and salt. Consider:

> **Baking:** Cooking food in a pan or dish surrounded by the hot, dry air of an oven. You can cook the food covered or uncovered. Baking generally doesn't require any added fat.

> **Broiling and grilling:** Both cooking methods expose food to direct heat.

To broil, place food on a broiler rack below a heating element.

To grill outdoors, place food on a grill rack above a bed of charcoal embers, or a gas flame. If you have an indoor grill, follow the manufacturer's directions. Both methods allow fat to drip away from the food.

> **Poaching:** This cooking technique gently simmers ingredients in water or a flavorful liquid, such as vinegar or broth, until cooked through and tender.

> **Roasting:** Like baking, roasting uses the oven's dry heat to cook the food. You can roast foods on a baking sheet or in a roasting pan. To maintain moisture, cook foods until they reach a safe internal temperature but don't overcook them.

> **Sautéing:** This method quickly cooks thin pieces of food. If use a good-quality nonstick pan, you can cook without added fat. For most recipes, you can use extra-virgin olive oil cooking spray or water in place of oil.

> **Stir-frying:** With this method, you quickly cook small, uniform-size pieces of food while rapidly stirring in a wok or large, nonstick skillet. You only need a small amount of oil or olive oil cooking spray.

> **Steaming:** This is one of the simplest and healthiest cooking techniques. It uses a perforated basket suspended over a simmering liquid. If you use a flavorful liquid or season the water, you'll flavor the food as it cooks. You can also steam in the microwave by placing the food in a microwave-safe dish and adding a small amount of water.

Ten Tips for Diabetic Success

1 **Educate yourself.** You will feel much more confident managing your diabetes if you arm yourself with the knowledge needed to take care of your health. Consider taking a healthy cooking class for inspiration, learn how to read food labels, or hire a personal trainer to jump-start your exercise program.

2 **Find your mantra.** Maria Robinson says, "Nobody can go back and start from the beginning, but anyone can start today and make a happy ending." Mantras both uplift you and keep you motivated. If work is difficult because food is always around or your coworkers or friends aren't supportive of your diabetes requirements, repeat your positive affirmation to keep you grounded.

3 **Plan ahead, even just one day.** If you set a goal to plan meals and snacks in advance, you won't be spontaneously tempted to choose unhealthy foods throughout the day. Planning will also ensure that you eat five servings of fruits and vegetables each day and stay within your carbohydrate goals.

4 **Go slowly.** Making positive changes to your diet and lifestyle will take time and setbacks will happen. Don't aim for perfection, rather focus on a little better, a little more. Don't let a splurge or missed exercise session become an excuse to give up. When you get off track, clean the slate and start fresh.

5 **Use the buddy system.** Finding other people with similar goals can greatly improve your success with diabetes management. Find a local diabetes support group to enlist help and learn while forming new friendships.

6 **Think of water as a food group.** Being dehydrated can cause tiredness, low energy, and headaches, and thirst is often mistaken for hunger. Carry a water bottle during the day and aim to drink at least eight 8-ounce glasses each day.

7 **Make exercise a daily habit.** Aim to be active for at least 10 minutes every day. Set your alarm 10 minutes earlier so you can walk around the block before you head to work. If you like TV, set up a treadmill in front of it so you can watch and walk. Think of exercise like you do brushing your teeth: do it every day.

8 **Eat mindfully.** Healthy eating is more than the food on your plate. It is also about how you think about food in general. Good eating habits can be learned. Slow down and think of food as nourishment rather than something to just gulp and run.

9 **Check portion sizes.** Even if you've been living with diabetes for years, check your portion know-how occasionally. Remember, carb amounts are based on specific serving sizes. So measure a serving of cereal or a 4-ounce glass of juice to see what a serving really looks like. Consider using smaller plates to keep portions in check.

10 **Create a healthy plate.** Fill half of your plate with colorful vegetables and fruits, one quarter with lean protein, and one quarter with high-fiber, unrefined complex carbohydrates. Eat more beans, dark green leafy vegetables, citrus fruits, sweet potatoes, berries, whole grains, fish high in omega-3 fats, nuts, and nonfat dairy products.

EXERCISE!

Exercise is one of the best things you can do to manage diabetes. Exercise helps your body use insulin, which controls your blood sugar. When you exercise, your muscles take up glucose for fuel. This helps lower blood-sugar levels. Exercise also helps you lose weight and maintain a healthy weight, lowers LDL or "bad" cholesterol, lowers blood sugar, strengthens muscles and bones, improves circulation, boosts energy and mood, lowers stress, decreases the risk for heart disease and stroke, and helps you sleep better.

Do check with your doctor before starting any new exercise program.

Don't think of exercise as a chore. Find something active that you like to do and add it to your day—just like you add healthy greens, blueberries, or salmon to your meals. Make a list of fun activities—you don't have to go to a gym to be active. Yoga, walking, swimming, and dancing are a few ideas. Any activity that raises your heart rate is good.

While exercising, carry a carbohydrate-containing snack, like fruit, in case your blood sugar gets low. If you haven't been active, start by incrementally increasing daily activities. For example, park your car farther from the store, take the stairs, walk to a coworker's desk rather than sending an e-mail, take a five-minute walk break every hour at work, cook more, and clean more! The benefits of lifelong exercise are abundant, so make it enjoyable and make it a habit.

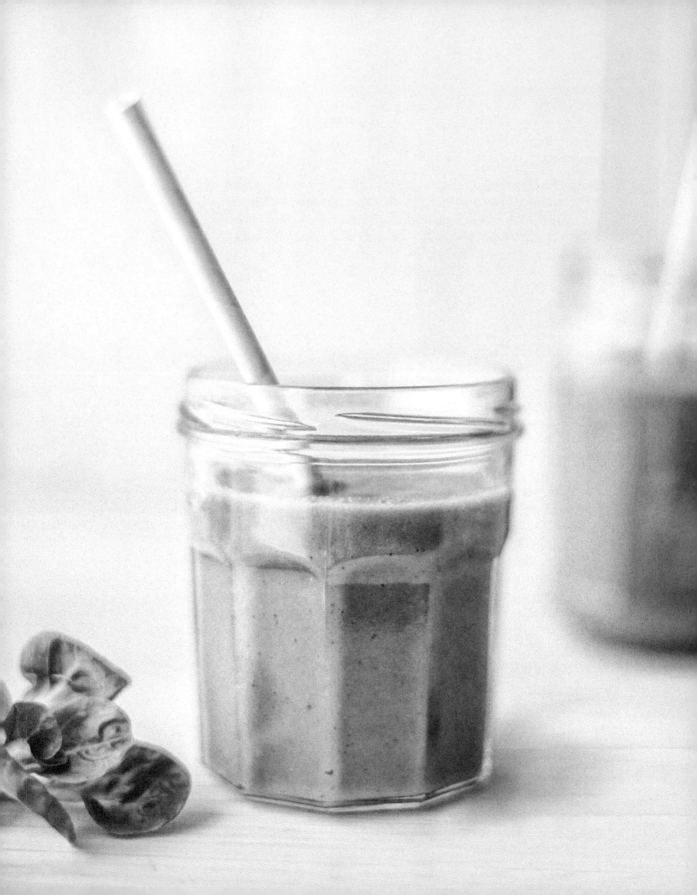

CHAPTER 3

Breakfast Bonanza

Baked Avocado and Egg

GLUTEN-FREE · QUICK & EASY
PREP TIME: 10 MINUTES · COOK TIME: 10 MINUTES

If you're trying to add variety to your diet while, at the same time, keep your blood-sugar levels in check, look no further than the mighty avocado. Despite this fruit's reputation for being high in calories and fat, the types of fat in avocados—omega-3s and oleic acid—are the types shown to lower the risk for cardiovascular disease. What's more, avocados are rich in soluble fiber and considered to be a low–glycemic index food that promotes blood-sugar regulation. They also have a wide range of anti-inflammatory benefits due to their high levels of antioxidants. Paired with protein-packed eggs and cottage cheese, this breakfast will keep you fueled and your blood sugar steady for hours.

1 large avocado, halved and pitted

2 large eggs

2 tomato slices, divided

½ cup nonfat cottage cheese, divided

Fresh cilantro, for garnish

1. Preheat the oven to 425°F.

2. Slice a thin piece from the bottom of each avocado half so they sit flat.

3. Remove a small amount from each avocado half to make a bigger hole to hold the egg.

4. On a small foil-lined baking sheet, place the halves hollow-side up.

5. Break 1 egg into each half.

6. Top each with 1 slice of tomato and ¼ cup of cottage cheese.

7. Place the sheet in the preheated oven. Bake for 8 to 10 minutes for softboiled consistency, or longer for a firmer egg.

8. Garnish with fresh cilantro and serve.

PER SERVING Calories: 275; Total Fat: 19g; Protein: 15g; Carbohydrates: 14g; Sugars: 5g; Fiber: 7g; Sodium: 306mg

RECIPE TIP: *This recipe also works well in a toaster oven. Consider making a double batch for a grab-and-go lunch or healthy snack.*

Lentil, Squash, and Tomato Omelet

GLUTEN-FREE

PREP TIME: 5 MINUTES • COOK TIME: 45 MINUTES

Lentils, a type of legume, are an absolute powerhouse of nutrition and an important food to include in any healthy meal plan. Lentils are a good source of cholesterol-lowering fiber that also prevents blood-sugar levels from rising too rapidly after a meal. They are also an excellent source of B vitamins, iron, and healthy-blood-pressure-promoting magnesium. This little bean is also quick cooking, in just about 20 minutes, making it a convenient source of protein—one cup of lentils has almost 18 grams of protein. That's more protein than two whole eggs!

1 cup water

⅓ cup dried lentils, picked over, rinsed, and drained

Extra-virgin olive oil cooking spray

1 medium zucchini, thinly sliced

½ cup grape tomatoes, coarsely chopped

1 garlic clove, chopped

2 tablespoons chopped fresh chives

2 large eggs

2 tablespoons nonfat milk

1. Preheat the oven to 350°F.

2. In a small saucepan set over high heat, heat the water until it boils.

3. Add the lentils. Reduce the heat to low. Simmer for about 15 minutes, or until most of the liquid has been absorbed. In a colander, drain and set aside.

4. Lightly coat an 8- or 9-inch nonstick skillet with cooking spray. Place the skillet over medium-high heat.

5. Add the zucchini, tomatoes, garlic, and chives. Sauté for 5 to 10 minutes, stirring frequently, or until soft.

6. Add the lentils to the skillet.

7. In a medium bowl, beat together the eggs and milk with a fork.

8. Lightly coat a small casserole or baking dish with cooking spray.

(continued)

9. In the bottom of the prepared dish, spread the vegetable mixture.

10. Pour the egg mixture over. Use a fork to distribute evenly.

11. Place the dish in the preheated oven. Bake for 15 to 20 minutes, or until the dish is set in the middle.

12. Slice in half and enjoy!

PER SERVING Calories: 181; Total Fat: 5g; Protein: 15g; Carbohydrates: 19g; Sugars 5g; Fiber: 9g; Sodium: 91mg

TOSS IT TOGETHER TIP: *Prepare a big batch of lentils and measure ½- and 1-cup portions. Store in the refrigerator or freezer. Use them when your meal needs a fiber and protein boost. You can toss them on salads and into soups, or use them in place of starchy carbs like potatoes. Cooked lentils combined with chopped sweet peppers make a delicious and nutritious cold salad that you can season with your favorite herbs and spices. Lentils can also be puréed and used in baked goods to increase the protein and fiber.*

Pumpkin–Peanut Butter Single-Serve Muffins

GLUTEN-FREE • DAIRY-FREE
PREP TIME: 10 MINUTES • COOK TIME: 25 MINUTES

Forget the snooze button! Antioxidant-rich pumpkin and powdered peanut butter pair with omega-3-rich flaxseed. These luscious, decadent-tasting single-serve muffins will have you racing out of bed to the breakfast table. Peanut butter is, no doubt, an excellent food to include in a diabetic diet due to its heart-healthy polyunsaturated fats and lack of cholesterol. But, for many people, peanut butter can be one of those things that is hard to eat moderately (taking a spoon to the jar does not count as moderate!). If that describes you, powdered peanut butter makes a great choice for maintaining the nutrition while keeping calories and total fat in check. This recipe is rich in protein, fiber, and slow-releasing carbohydrates.

2 tablespoons powdered peanut butter

2 tablespoons coconut flour

2 tablespoons finely ground flaxseed

1 teaspoon pumpkin pie spice

½ teaspoon baking powder

1 tablespoon dried cranberries

½ cup water

1 cup canned pumpkin

2 large eggs

½ teaspoon vanilla extract

Extra-virgin olive oil cooking spray

1. Preheat the oven to 350°F.

2. In a medium bowl, stir together the powdered peanut butter, coconut flour, flaxseed, pumpkin pie spice, baking powder, dried cranberries, and water.

3. In a separate medium bowl, whisk together the pumpkin and eggs until smooth.

4. Add the pumpkin mixture to the dry ingredients. Stir to combine.

5. Add the vanilla. Mix together well.

6. Spray 2 (8-ounce) ramekins with cooking spray.

(continued)

7. Spoon half of the batter into each ramekin.

8. Place the ramekins on a baking and carefully transfer the sheet to the preheated oven. Bake for 25 minutes, or until a toothpick in the center comes out clean. Enjoy immediately!

PER SERVING Calories: 219; Total Fat: 9g; Protein: 13g; Carbohydrates: 24g; Sugars: 9g; Fiber: 10g; Sodium: 137mg

NOTE: *You can also microwave the ramekins, one at a time, for about 2 minutes on high, or until firm.*

INGREDIENT TIP: *Powdered peanut butter is sold in most grocery stores with brand names such as PB2 and PBFit. You can also buy defatted peanut flour, which is the same thing, from online retailers like Amazon. Powdered peanut butter can be reconstituted and used in any dish that calls for regular peanut butter, including on sandwiches, in smoothies, and on fruit. Keep a couple of jars in your pantry and get creative!*

Creamy Blueberry Quesadillas

QUICK & EASY

PREP TIME: 5 MINUTES • COOK TIME: 5 MINUTES

Quesadillas may not be what you typically think of as a breakfast food when following a diabetic food plan. However, this one has had a low-carb makeover with the use of ready-made whole-grain, high-fiber, low-carb tortillas, and a high-protein filling of ricotta cheese and Greek yogurt. The flaxseed boosts the soluble-fiber content and adds heart-healthy omega-3 fats. Antioxidant-rich blueberries replace sugar-filled jams for an extra nutritional punch. Vary the berries to suit your taste and enjoy!

¼ cup plain nonfat
    Greek yogurt

¼ cup nonfat ricotta cheese

2 tablespoons finely
    ground flaxseed

½ teaspoon cinnamon

¼ teaspoon vanilla extract

1 tablespoon granulated stevia

2 (8-inch) low-carb whole-
    wheat tortillas

½ cup fresh
    blueberries, divided

1. Preheat the oven to 400°F.

2. Line a baking dish with aluminum foil.

3. In a small bowl, mix together the yogurt, ricotta cheese, flaxseed, cinnamon, vanilla, and stevia.

4. Place the tortillas in the baking dish.

5. Spread half of the yogurt mixture on each tortilla, almost to the edges.

6. Top each with ¼ cup of blueberries. Fold the tortillas in half.

7. Place the dish in the preheated oven. Bake for 3 to 4 minutes.

8. Enjoy immediately!

PER SERVING Calories: 159; Total Fat: 6g; Protein: 12g; Carbohydrates: 21g; Sugars: 6g; Fiber: 10g; Sodium: 223mg

RECIPE TIP: *This recipe can also be prepared in a toaster oven. Whole-grain, low-carb tortillas are an essential pantry item for diabetic cooking. Very low in carbs, yet high in fiber and protein, low-carb tortillas make it easy to enjoy old favorites like burritos and sandwich wraps. They also make a great substitute for carb-laden pizza dough and can be baked into healthy, homemade low-carb tortilla chips.*

Grain-Free Applesauce Crêpes

QUICK & EASY

PREP TIME: 5 MINUTES · COOK TIME: 10 MINUTES

You won't miss the white flour in these grain-free crêpes. Coconut flour has gone mainstream due to its numerous health benefits, great taste, and light texture. Coconut flour is gluten-free and can be used in place of white or wheat flour in recipes for a lower-carb, higher-fiber product. With five grams of fiber per tablespoon, coconut flour helps keep you feeling full and promotes healthy digestion. The fiber in coconut flour doesn't spike your blood sugar like refined grained-based flours—definitely a benefit for managing blood-sugar levels. This recipe may take a bit of practice, but you are certain to impress when you serve these low-carb, high-protein crêpes at your next brunch!

½ cup liquid egg substitute

½ cup coconut flour

¾ cup unsweetened vanilla almond milk

1 teaspoon vanilla extract

1 teaspoon granulated stevia

Pinch salt

Extra-virgin olive oil cooking spray

½ cup unsweetened applesauce

½ cup nonfat cottage cheese

Ground cinnamon

1. To a blender, add the egg substitute, coconut flour, vanilla almond milk, vanilla, stevia, and salt. Process until thoroughly mixed.

2. Place a nonstick skillet set over medium-high heat. Coat with cooking spray.

3. When the pan is hot, pour in a one-half of the batter. Swirl to evenly coat the bottom of the pan. Cook for about 2 minutes, or until the top is set and the bottom is light brown.

4. Using a silicone spatula, loosen the top edge of the crêpe. Tilting the pan, roll the crêpe toward the bottom of the pan. Remove from the pan and set aside. Repeat with the remaining batter.

5. In a small, covered microwave-safe bowl, gently warm the applesauce in the microwave on medium for about 30 seconds.

6. Remove from the microwave. Add the cottage cheese. Mix gently until blended.

7. Divide the crêpes between 2 plates.

8. Top each with ½ cup of the applesauce–cottage cheese mixture.

9. Sprinkle with cinnamon and serve immediately.

PER SERVING Calories: 200; Total Fat: 5g; Protein: 21g; Carbohydrates: 33g; Sugars: 14g; Fiber: 17g; Sodium: 455mg

NOTE: *Tightly wrapped crêpes can be refrigerated for 3 days or frozen for later use. Add your favorite filling and serve. This recipe can also be prepared in a toaster oven.*

INGREDIENT TIP: *Keep coconut flour on hand as a pantry staple. Use it in pancakes and other baked goods, to replace half or all of the bread crumbs in meatloaf, and as a substitute for grains when making gravies and breading for fish and meats. Coconut flour absorbs a lot of liquid, so you will have to make slight adjustments to your recipes by increasing the amount of liquid.*

Goji Berry Muesli

PREP TIME: 10 MINUTES • CHILLING TIME: 8 HOURS, OR OVERNIGHT

This traditional Swiss breakfast cereal is a nice change come spring and summer after a long winter of hot oatmeal. The variations are endless—use any fruit or nut you like. The nonfat Greek yogurt boosts the protein content so you stay fuller longer; the nuts and seeds add heart-healthy fats and fiber. Considered both a fruit and an herb, goji berries are typically found in Asian and European countries, but they have hit the United States and can be found in most grocery stores. Goji berries are an excellent source of antioxidants, and are low in calories and high in fiber. There is some evidence that goji berries can interact with certain drugs. If you take warfarin, simply replace the goji berries with your favorite dried fruit.

½ cup old-fashioned rolled oats

½ cup plain nonfat Greek yogurt

2 tablespoons dried goji berries, or dried blueberries, cherries, or cranberries

1 teaspoon liquid stevia

½ teaspoon vanilla extract

½ cup fresh blueberries, divided

3 teaspoons pumpkin seeds, divided

3 teaspoons finely ground flaxseed, divided

½ cup unsweetened vanilla almond milk, divided

1. In a medium bowl, stir together the oats, yogurt, goji berries, stevia, and vanilla.

2. Evenly divide the mixture between 2 small bowls. Cover and refrigerate overnight.

3. The next morning, top each serving with ¼ cup of blueberries, 1½ teaspoons of pumpkin seeds, and 1½ teaspoons of flaxseed. Stir to combine. Let sit for 5 to 10 minutes.

4. Top each with ¼ cup of vanilla almond milk and enjoy cold!

PER SERVING Calories: 230; Total Fat: 7g; Protein: 13g; Carbohydrates: 30g; Sugars: 9g; Fiber: 4g; Sodium: 70mg

RECIPE TIP: *Cover and refrigerate for up to 1 day. You can eat the muesli cold, or warm it in the microwave.*

TOSS IT TOGETHER TIP: *Store leftover nuts and seeds in the freezer to keep them fresh. Let sit on the counter for a few minutes to thaw before using. Flaxseed can be used on just about anything—from smoothies to salads to steamed vegetables. The type of fiber in flaxseed can lower bad cholesterol and increase your feeling of fullness, which means you may eat less food—a bonus for anyone trying to lose weight. Look for finely ground flaxseed; the whole seeds will just pass through you without being digested, making for a good laxative if needed.*

Cinnamon-Almond Green Smoothie

PREP TIME: 4 MINUTES

Smoothies are one of the fastest meals on the planet. There are endless combinations you can throw together for a meal-in-a-glass packed with protein, healthy fats, fiber, slow-releasing carbs, and nutrient-rich fruits and vegetables. All you need is a decent blender and a few core ingredients, so let the blender be your canvas! This diabetic-friendly recipe uses high-protein Greek yogurt and a combination of antioxidant and soluble fiber–rich spinach and apples. A healthy dose of heart-healthy fats is provided by the almond butter and flaxseed, and finished off with blood sugar–balancing cinnamon.

1½ cups nonfat milk

2 tablespoons finely ground flaxseed

1 tablespoon almond butter

1 (8-ounce) container plain nonfat Greek yogurt

1 cup frozen spinach

1 small apple, peeled, cored, and finely chopped

1 teaspoon vanilla extract

1 teaspoon cinnamon

Stevia, for sweetening

4 to 6 ice cubes (optional)

1. In a blender, combine the milk, flaxseed, and almond butter. Blend for 10 seconds on medium.

2. Add the yogurt, spinach, apple, vanilla, cinnamon, stevia, and ice cubes (if using). Blend for about 1 minute, or until smooth and creamy.

3. Pour into 2 glasses and sip to your health!

PER SERVING Calories: 278; Total Fat: 8g; Protein: 24g; Carbohydrates: 21g; Sugars: 15g; Fiber: 6g, Sodium: 185mg

TOSS IT TOGETHER TIP: *Store almond butter in the refrigerator to increase its shelf life. Consider using almond butter and a sprinkle of cinnamon and granulated stevia on toast in place of sugar-filled jellies and jams for a healthier alternative.*

Peach Pancakes

GLUTEN-FREE • QUICK & EASY
PREP TIME: 5 MINUTES • COOK TIME: 15 MINUTES

Who said a diabetic diet can't include pancakes? All it takes is a little recipe magic and pancakes are back on the menu! High-fiber, slow-digesting coconut flour lowers the carb content of these delicious pancakes while increasing the protein content. Low–glycemic index peaches and nutrient-rich pumpkin start your day with some recommended fruit and vegetable servings. Peaches contain vitamins A and C, potassium, and fiber. Pumpkin is rich in vitamins A, C, E, beta-carotene, and antioxidants. Both make these high-protein pancakes a great choice for managing blood-sugar levels.

1 medium peach, finely diced

⅓ cup coconut flour

½ cup nonfat cottage cheese

½ cup canned pumpkin

½ cup unsweetened almond milk

2 tablespoons chia seeds

1 teaspoon vanilla extract

1 teaspoon baking powder

⅛ teaspoon salt

1 teaspoon cinnamon

1 to 2 teaspoons granulated stevia

4 large egg whites, beaten

Extra-virgin olive oil cooking spray

Sugar-free maple syrup, for serving

1. In a small bowl, mix together the peach, coconut flour, cottage cheese, pumpkin, almond milk, chia seeds, vanilla, baking powder, salt, cinnamon, and stevia.

2. Add the egg whites. Stir until thoroughly combined.

3. Spray a nonstick skillet with cooking spray. Place it over medium-high heat for 1 to 2 minutes, or until completely preheated. The first pancake should cook thoroughly.

4. In the skillet, drop about 2 tablespoons of batter for each silver dollar-size pancake. Cook for 2 to 3 minutes on each side, or until golden. Transfer to a plate. Repeat with the remaining batter, re-spraying the skillet with cooking spray between each batch.

5. Top with your favorite sugar-free syrup and devour immediately!

PER SERVING Calories: 251; Total Fat: 8g; Protein: 25g; Carbohydrates: 33g; Sugars: 14g; Fiber: 18g; Sodium: 409mg

RECIPE TIP: *When making these pancakes, don't expect them to be light and fluffy. The cottage cheese and pumpkin make them denser, and the batter is thicker than a traditional pancake batter. They won't bubble like traditional pancakes either, so watch that they cook thoroughly without burning.*

Veggie and Tofu Scramble

DAIRY-FREE • QUICK & EASY
PREP TIME: 5 MINUTES • COOK TIME: 10 MINUTES

Scrambled tofu makes an excellent dairy-free, cholesterol-free, saturated fat-free, and high-protein alternative to scrambled eggs. Tofu, also known as bean curd, is made by coagulating soy milk and pressing it into blocks. Tofu has a bland, subtle flavor and easily takes on the flavors of the herbs and spices used to season it. Tofu is sold in various forms including soft, firm, and extra firm. Soft tofu is best for smoothies and puddings, while firm and extra firm are best for stir-frying, baking, and scrambling. You can basically do anything with tofu—so be bold and have fun! Try scrambling some tofu for your next breakfast, lunch, or dinner.

1 pound firm- or extra-firm tofu

1 teaspoon dry mustard

1 teaspoon ground cumin

1 tablespoon extra-virgin olive oil

2 medium tomatoes, diced

1 medium zucchini, chopped

¾ cup sliced fresh mushrooms

2 garlic cloves, minced

1 bunch spinach, rinsed and chopped

½ teaspoon low-sodium soy sauce

1 teaspoon freshly squeezed lemon juice

Freshly ground black pepper

1. In a colander, drain the tofu.

2. In a medium bowl, crumble the drained tofu.

3. Add the mustard and cumin. Toss until well mixed.

4. In a nonstick skillet set over medium-high heat, heat the olive oil.

5. Add the tomatoes, zucchini, mushrooms, and garlic. Sauté for 2 to 3 minutes. Reduce the heat to medium-low.

6. Add the spinach, tofu, soy sauce, and lemon juice.

7. Cover and cook for 5 to 7 minutes, stirring occasionally.

8. Season with pepper and serve immediately.

PER SERVING Calories: 348; Total Fat: 18g; Protein: 29g; Carbohydrates: 25g; Sugars: 3g; Fiber: 11g; Sodium: 220mg

INGREDIENT TIP: *Consider picking up some Bragg Liquid Aminos to use in place of traditional soy sauce. Bragg, made from soybeans, is gluten-free and contains less sodium then even low-sodium varieties of soy sauce.*

Very Cherry Overnight Oatmeal in a Jar

PREP TIME: 5 MINUTES, PLUS 5 HOURS CHILLING TIME, OR OVERNIGHT

This breakfast is a complete meal in a glass containing foods from all food groups. Once you master this recipe, it is sure to become a go-to breakfast favorite. Use mason jars for perfect portion control. Chia seeds make this recipe nice and thick and provide soluble fiber and omega-3 fats. Sweet and tart cherries are high in anthocyanins—a powerful antioxidant. They also contain a naturally occurring chemical that may help lower blood-sugar levels in diabetics. Check the ingredients in your cherries and make certain they don't contain any added sugars.

½ cup uncooked old-fashioned rolled oats

½ cup nonfat milk

½ cup plain nonfat Greek yogurt

2 tablespoons chia seeds

1 teaspoon liquid stevia

1 teaspoon cinnamon

½ teaspoon vanilla extract

½ cup frozen cherries, divided

1. In a small bowl, mix together the oats, milk, yogurt, chia seeds, stevia, cinnamon, and vanilla.

2. Evenly divide the oat mixture between 2 mason jars or individual containers. Cover tightly and shake until well combined.

3. To each jar, stir in ¼ cup of cherries.

4. Seal the containers and refrigerate overnight.

5. The next day, enjoy chilled or heated.

PER SERVING Calories: 218; Total Fat: 5g; Protein: 14g; Carbohydrates: 29g; Sugars: 10g; Fiber: 5g; Sodium: 54mg

RECIPE TIP: *This oatmeal can be kept refrigerated for 3 days. It makes breakfast quick, easy, and portable. Make several at once and enjoy throughout the work week. This recipe is also great with leftover grains from other meals, like quinoa, millet, tapioca, or other breakfast flakes like spelt and barley. For extra fiber or to use up supplies, increase the amount of chia seeds or substitute flaxseed for a nutty flavor.*

Mandarin Orange–Millet Breakfast Bowl

GLUTEN-FREE

PREP TIME: 5 MINUTES • COOK TIME: 30 MINUTES

Millet is a tiny round seed that, if you don't know already, you may want to become familiar with for its heart-protecting properties and high mineral content. Creamy like mashed potatoes or fluffy like rice, millet is a delicious grain used in both sweet and savory dishes. Millet's high fiber content slows digestion and releases sugar into the bloodstream at a more even rate. It is also high in magnesium, a mineral involved in the body's use of glucose and insulin secretion. Millet can be white, gray, red, or yellow and is widely available in the grain section of most grocery stores.

⅓ cup millet

1 cup nonfat milk

½ cup water

¼ teaspoon cinnamon

¼ teaspoon
    ground cardamom

1 teaspoon vanilla extract

Pinch salt

Stevia, for sweetening

½ cup canned mandarin
    oranges, drained

2 tablespoons sliced almonds

1. In a small saucepan set over medium-high heat, stir together the millet, milk, water, cinnamon, cardamom, vanilla, salt, and stevia. Bring to a boil. Reduce the heat to low. Cover and simmer for 25 minutes, without stirring. If the liquid is not completely absorbed, cook for 3 to 5 minutes longer, partially covered.

2. Stir in the oranges. Remove from the heat.

3. Top with the sliced almonds and serve.

PER SERVING Calories: 215; Total Fat: 4g; Protein: 9g; Carbohydrates: 37g; Sugars: 12g; Fiber: 4g; Sodium: 62mg

TOSS IT TOGETHER TIP: *Toss cooked and chilled millet with your favorite chopped vegetables, grilled chicken, or baked tofu cubes. Season as desired and dinner is served! To impart a nuttier flavor to cooked millet, toast the grains before cooking. To do this, place the grains in a dry skillet over medium heat and stir frequently. When they turn a golden color, add them to the boiling cooking liquid. Millet can also be ground and added to bread and muffin recipes.*

Quinoa Breakfast Bake with Pistachios and Plums

GLUTEN-FREE

PREP TIME: 10 MINUTES • COOK TIME: 1 HOUR

Quinoa is unique among grains because it contains all of the essential amino acids your body needs, making it a source of high-quality complete protein. Quinoa cooks quickly, in about 15 minutes, and its distinctive nut-like flavor tastes great too! It can be found in the grain aisle of grocery stores or in bulk bins. Quinoa creates the base of this tasty baked breakfast, along with vitamin- and mineral-rich pistachios and plums. Baked in mini loaf pans, this is a perfect breakfast for two!

Extra-virgin olive oil cooking spray

⅓ cup dry quinoa, thoroughly rinsed

1 teaspoon vanilla extract

1 teaspoon cinnamon

½ teaspoon nutmeg

Stevia, for sweetening

2 large egg whites

1 cup nonfat milk

2 plums, chopped, divided

4 tablespoons chopped unsalted pistachios, divided

1. Preheat the oven to 350°F.

2. Spray two mini loaf pans with cooking spray. Set aside.

3. In a medium bowl, stir together the quinoa, vanilla, cinnamon, nutmeg, and stevia until the quinoa is coated with the spices.

4. Pour half of the quinoa mixture into each loaf pan.

5. In the same medium bowl, beat the egg whites and thoroughly whisk in the milk.

6. Evenly scatter half of the plums and 2 tablespoons of pistachios in each pan.

7. Pour half of the egg mixture over each loaf. Stir lightly to partially submerge the plums.

8. Place the pans in the preheated oven. Bake for 1 hour, or until the loaves are set, with only a small amount of liquid remaining.

9. Remove from the pans and enjoy hot!

PER SERVING Calories: 230; Total Fat: 5g; Protein: 13g; Carbohydrates: 38g; Sugars: 12g; Fiber: 6g; Sodium: 155mg

TOSS IT TOGETHER TIP: *Toss together quinoa with rinsed, canned pinto beans, pumpkin seeds, scallions, and coriander for a south-of-the-border-inspired meal.*

Mini Spinach–Broccoli Quiches

GLUTEN-FREE
PREP TIME: 5 MINUTES • COOK TIME: 35 MINUTES

When cooking for two people, there is nothing easier than throwing together a few simple ingredients, tossing them into a ramekin, pouring an egg on top, and baking for half an hour. Mini crustless quiches are simple to prepare in small quantities and homey, unlike that cold cereal for breakfast. The spinach and broccoli add cholesterol-lowering fiber, vitamins, minerals, and antioxidants, and more than two servings of vegetables per recipe! Broccoli is one cruciferous vegetable you will want to include in your diet on a regular basis for its potent cardiovascular and anti-cancer benefits.

Extra-virgin olive oil
   cooking spray
1 cup frozen broccoli florets
½ cup frozen spinach
2 large eggs
2 large egg whites
¼ cup unsweetened almond
   milk, or nonfat dairy milk
Salt, to season
Freshly ground black pepper,
   to season
2 tablespoons fresh
   dill, divided
Shredded nonfat cheese, for
   garnish (optional)

1. Preheat the oven to 400°F.

2. Spray two (8-ounce) ramekins with cooking spray.

3. In a small microwave-safe dish, mix together the broccoli and spinach. Place in the microwave and thaw on high for 30 seconds. Remove from the microwave and drain off any excess liquid.

4. Fill each ramekin with half of the vegetable mixture.

5. In a medium bowl, beat the eggs and egg whites with the almond milk. Season with salt and pepper.

6. Evenly divide the egg mixture between the ramekins.

7. Top each with 1 tablespoon of dill. Garnish with the shredded cheese (if using).

8. Place the ramekins on a baking sheet. Carefully transfer the sheet to the preheated oven. Bake for about 35 minutes, or until the center is firm and the top is golden brown.

PER SERVING Calories: 117; Total Fat: 1g; Protein: 11g; Carbohydrates: 3g; Sugars: 1g; Fiber: 1g; Sodium: 191mg

RECIPE TIP: *Make a double batch and take a mini quiche to work for lunch.*

White Bean–Oat Waffles

DAIRY-FREE • QUICK & EASY
PREP TIME: 10 MINUTES • COOK TIME: 20 MINUTES

All beans are considered low–glycemic index foods, but cannellini beans are one of the lowest. They are digested slowly, providing steady energy and stabilizing blood-sugar levels for hours. Cannellini beans, also known as white kidney beans, are rich in fiber, magnesium, iron, and folate, and are very versatile with an indescribable nutty flavor. But beans in a waffle? Beans give this traditionally high-carb dish a makeover by boosting the protein and increasing the overall nutrient content. The batter is made with a combination of slow-digesting oats and fiber-filled flaxseed. Top with fresh fruit or unsweetened applesauce and enjoy the yummy wholesomeness of these delicious waffles!

1 large egg white

2 tablespoons finely ground flaxseed

½ cup water

¼ teaspoon salt

1 teaspoon vanilla extract

½ cup cannellini beans, drained and rinsed

1 teaspoon coconut oil

1 teaspoon liquid stevia

½ cup old-fashioned rolled oats

Extra-virgin olive oil cooking spray

1. In a blender, combine the egg white, flaxseed, water, salt, vanilla, cannellini beans, coconut oil, and stevia. Blend on high for 90 seconds.

2. Add the oats. Blend for 1 minute more.

3. Preheat the waffle iron. The batter will thicken to the correct consistency while the waffle iron preheats.

4. Spray the heated waffle iron with cooking spray.

5. Add ¾ cup of batter. Close the waffle iron. Cook for 6 to 8 minutes, or until done. Repeated with the remaining batter.

6. Serve hot, with your favorite sugar-free topping.

PER SERVING Calories: 169; Total Fat: 4g; Protein: 9g; Carbohydrates: 26g; Sugars: 1g; Fiber: 7g; Sodium: 165mg

TOSS IT TOGETHER TIP: *Store leftover beans in ½-cup portions and refrigerate or freeze them for later use. Cannellini beans can be used as a side for dinner, thrown in a quick breakfast burrito, tossed on salads, or mixed with leftover grains, steamed vegetables, and chicken, fish, or tofu for a healthy meal in minutes. Beans can also be added to smoothies for extra thickening power and to increase the protein content.*

Black Bean Breakfast Burrito

QUICK & EASY
PREP TIME: 10 MINUTES • COOK TIME: 10 MINUTES

This super-fast, nutritious breakfast can be put together in minutes using canned black beans and low-carb whole-wheat tortillas. One cup of black beans has nearly 15 grams of fiber and 15 grams of protein. This health-supportive mix of protein plus fiber is a great alternative to sodium- and saturated fat–filled breakfast meats. Outstanding for their support in managing blood sugar, black beans also keep the digestive tract running smoothly and your heart healthy.

Extra-virgin olive oil cooking spray

½ cup chopped onion

½ cup chopped bell pepper, any color

1 cup canned black beans, drained and rinsed

1 cup finely chopped fresh kale, thoroughly washed

1 teaspoon ground cumin

1 teaspoon freshly squeezed lime juice

2 (7-inch) low-carb whole-wheat tortillas

½ avocado, sliced, divided

4 tablespoons salsa, divided

Shredded nonfat cheese, for garnish (optional)

1. Spray a medium skillet with cooking oil. Place it over medium-high heat.

2. Add the onion and bell pepper. Sauté for 3 minutes.

3. Add the black beans, kale, cumin, and lime juice. Stir to combine. Reduce the heat to medium low. Cover and simmer for 5 minutes.

4. Top each tortilla with half of the avocado slices and 2 tablespoons of salsa.

5. Remove the bean mixture from the heat. Evenly divide it between the tortillas.

6. Garnish with the cheese (if using) and enjoy immediately!

PER SERVING Calories: 265; Total Fat: 10g; Protein: 15g; Carbohydrates: 40g; Sugars: 17g; Fiber: 17g; Sodium: 280mg

TOSS IT TOGETHER TIP: *Refrigerate or freeze leftover beans in ½-cup portions and use them as a topping for sweet potatoes, to make soup, and on salads. Make a bean bowl for one by layering black beans, avocado slices, chopped tomatoes, and diced onions. Top with fresh cilantro and shredded nonfat cheese.*

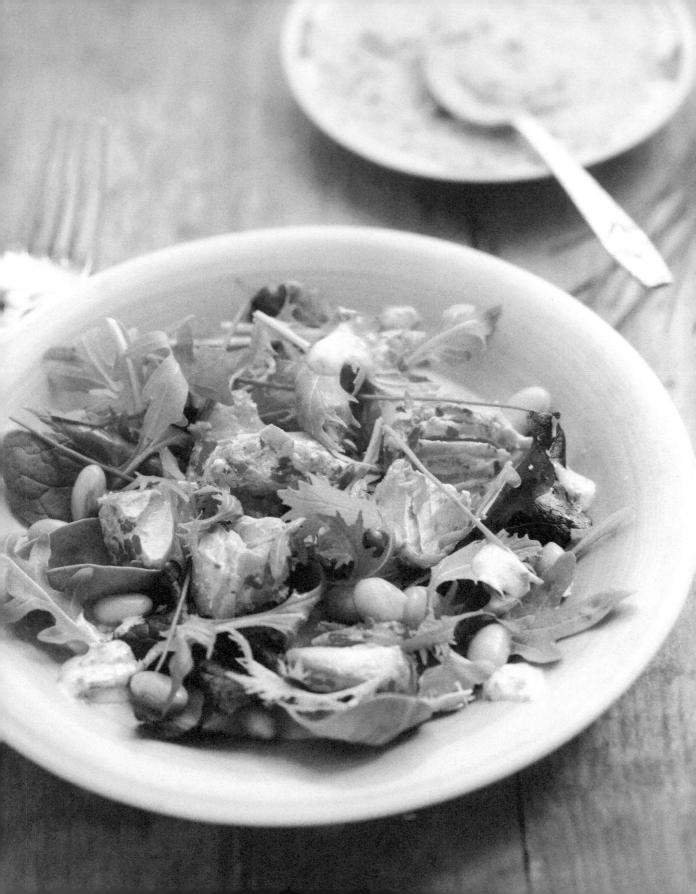

Meal-Size Salads

Edamame and Walnut Salad

GLUTEN-FREE · DAIRY-FREE · QUICK & EASY
PREP TIME: 10 MINUTES

Unique among nuts, walnuts contain the highest amounts of plant-based omega-3 essential fatty acids, which have beneficial effects on cardiovascular health and promote healthy blood pressure. Walnuts are also rich in antioxidants, protein, fiber, magnesium, vitamin B_6, and phosphorus. California grows more than 35 varieties and they display various shades—from light to amber— depending on the region in which they are grown. Tossed with high-protein edamame and a ginger Dijon vinaigrette, this mix is served on a bed of vitamin- and mineral-rich spinach.

For the vinaigrette

2 tablespoons
    balsamic vinegar

1 tablespoon extra-virgin
    olive oil

1 teaspoon grated fresh ginger

½ teaspoon Dijon mustard

Pinch salt

Freshly ground black pepper,
    to season

For the salad

1 cup shelled edamame

½ cup shredded carrots

½ cup shredded red cabbage

½ cup walnut halves

6 cups prewashed baby
    spinach, divided

To make the vinaigrette

In a small bowl, whisk together the balsamic vinegar, olive oil, ginger, Dijon mustard, and salt. Season with pepper. Set aside.

To make the salad

1. In a medium bowl, mix together the edamame, carrots, red cabbage, and walnuts.

2. Add the vinaigrette. Toss to coat.

3. Place 3 cups of spinach on each of 2 serving plates.

4. Top each serving with half of the dressed vegetables.

5. Enjoy immediately!

PER SERVING Calories: 426; Total Fat: 27g; Protein: 20g; Carbohydrates: 27g; Sugars: 8g; Fiber: 6g; Sodium: 168mg

TOSS IT TOGETHER TIP: *Make your own pesto with leftover walnuts. In a food processor, blend together fresh basil, walnuts, extra-virgin olive oil, and garlic. Serve on whole-grain bread, tossed with whole-grain pasta, or mixed with grains. Chopped walnuts also make a great addition to hot and cold breakfast cereals, mixed into yogurt and smoothies, or processed into homemade walnut butter.*

Quinoa, Beet, and Greens Salad

GLUTEN-FREE • DAIRY-FREE

PREP TIME: 15 MINUTES, PLUS 1 HOUR CHILLING TIME • COOK TIME: 25 MINUTES

This plant-powered, quick, and wholesome salad uses high-protein quinoa and roasted soy nuts to create a nutty, crunchy meal that is sure to please. Soy nuts are high in isoflavones, a type of phytochemical shown in hundreds of studies to help prevent heart disease and certain types of cancer. Soy nuts are lower in calories and fat, and higher in protein and fiber than other nuts. A one-quarter-cup serving has about 120 calories, 10 grams of protein, and 6 grams of fiber. Fiber- and potassium-rich beets are mixed in for their beneficial effects on reducing insulin resistance.

For the vinaigrette

1 tablespoon extra-virgin olive oil

2 tablespoons red wine vinegar

1 garlic clove, chopped

Freshly ground black pepper, to season

For the salad

2 medium beets

1 small bunch fresh kale leaves, thoroughly washed, deveined, and dried

Extra-virgin olive oil cooking spray

⅓ cup dry quinoa

⅔ cup water

¼ cup chopped scallions

½ cup unsalted soy nuts

To make the vinaigrette

In a large bowl, whisk together the olive oil, red wine vinegar, and garlic. Season with pepper. Set aside.

To make the salad

1. Into a medium saucepan set over high heat, insert a steamer basket. Fill the pan with water to just below the bottom of the steamer. Cover and bring to a boil.

2. Add the beets. Cover and steam for 7 to 10 minutes, or until just tender. Remove from the steamer. Let sit until cool enough to handle. Peel and slice. Set aside.

3. Spray the kale leaves with cooking spray. Massage the leaves, breaking down the fibers so they're easier to chew. Chop finely. You should have 1 cup.

4. In a small saucepan set over high heat, mix together the quinoa and water. Bring to a boil. Reduce the heat to medium-low. Cover and simmer for about 15 minutes, or until the quinoa is tender and the liquid has been absorbed. Remove from the heat.

(continued)

5. Immediately add half of the vinaigrette to the saucepan while fluffing the quinoa with a fork. Cover and refrigerate for at least 1 hour, or until completely cooled. Set aside the remaining vinaigrette.

6. Into the cooled quinoa, stir the chopped kale, scallions, soy nuts, sliced beets, and remaining vinaigrette. Toss lightly before serving.

PER SERVING Calories: 357; Total Fat: 16g; Protein: 16g; Carbohydrates: 38g; Sugars: 6g; Fiber: 9g; Sodium: 166mg

TOSS IT TOGETHER TIP: *Soy nuts are sold in bulk bins. Paired with other nuts, they make an excellent snack. Pair ¼ cup with half an apple—you'll have a low-carb, high-fiber, high-protein diabetic-friendly snack to keep your blood sugar steady between lunch and dinner. Homemade soy nuts are easy to make, too! You can soak and cook soybeans or used canned to reduce prep time. Simply bake them in a 350°F oven for about 45 minutes.*

Romaine Lettuce Salad with Cranberry, Feta, and Beans

GLUTEN-FREE • QUICK & EASY
PREP TIME: 10 MINUTES

This salad contains fat-free feta cheese to keep the tangy, powerful flavor while eliminating the unhealthy saturated fat and cholesterol. High in protein, calcium, and vitamin D, it only takes a small amount of feta to add flavor to dishes. The green beans and kidney beans complete the Greek theme, with an added touch of sweet and tart from antioxidant-rich dried cranberries. The phytonutrients in cranberries have been shown to protect against urinary tract infections, and provide powerful anti-inflammatory properties that support the immune system and decrease risks for developing cardiovascular disease and certain types of cancer.

1 cup chopped fresh
   green beans

6 cups washed and chopped
   romaine lettuce

1 cup sliced radishes

2 scallions, sliced

¼ cup chopped fresh oregano

1 cup canned kidney beans,
   drained and rinsed

½ cup cranberries, fresh
   or frozen

¼ cup crumbled fat-free
   feta cheese

1 tablespoon extra-virgin
   olive oil

Salt, to season

Freshly ground black pepper,
   to season

1. In a microwave-safe dish, add the green beans and a small amount of water. Microwave on high for about 2 minutes, or until tender.

2. In a large bowl, toss together the romaine lettuce, radishes, scallions, and oregano.

3. Add the green beans, kidney beans, cranberries, feta cheese, and olive oil. Season with salt and pepper. Toss to coat.

4. Evenly divide between 2 plates and enjoy immediately.

PER SERVING Calories: 283; Total Fat: 9g; Protein: 17g; Carbohydrates: 42g; Sugars: 10g; Fiber: 13g; Sodium: 612mg

TOSS IT TOGETHER TIP: *You can usually find fresh cranberries year-round in most produce departments, or in the freezer section. Cranberries are very low in calories and can be mixed into breakfast cereals and baked into savory dishes. Cranberries are considered to be a medium–glycemic index food, so they fit with a diabetic meal plan. You can also toss together leftover grains, kidney beans, feta, cranberries, and fresh mint using a simple formula of: grain + bean + feta + berry + herb. Just add your favorite dressing and enjoy!*

Chickpea "Tuna" Salad

GLUTEN-FREE • QUICK & EASY
PREP TIME: 15 MINUTES

Traditional tuna salad can be high in calories and unhealthy saturated fat and cholesterol because it is typically made with mayonnaise. This wonderfully simple, tasty recipe is a mock tuna salad made with chickpeas. Great alone or on a bed of romaine lettuce or baby greens, this dish is healthy and wholesome. It won't taste exactly like tuna fish, but it will give you the mouthfeel and satisfaction of its unhealthy cousin.

2 cups canned chickpeas, drained and rinsed

½ cup plain nonfat Greek yogurt

2 small celery stalks, chopped

1 small cucumber, chopped

½ cup chopped red onion

2 tablespoons freshly squeezed lemon juice

1 tablespoon chia seeds

1 garlic clove, chopped

1 teaspoon minced fresh parsley

Salt, to season

Freshly ground black pepper, to season

2 large romaine lettuce leaves

1. In a medium bowl, roughly mash the chickpeas with the back of a fork.

2. Add the yogurt, celery, cucumber, red onion, lemon juice, chia seeds, garlic, and parsley. Mix well. Season with salt and pepper.

3. Place half of the chickpea mixture on each romaine lettuce leaf. Wrap and serve chilled or at room temperature.

PER SERVING Calories: 283; Total Fat: 7g; Protein: 19g; Carbohydrates: 39g; Sugars: 2g; Fiber: 15g; Sodium: 70mg

RECIPE TIP: *An optional ingredient to add here is crushed nori or dulse. Nori and dulse are types of seaweed that are dried or toasted. Nori is sold in sheets and used as the wrapping for sushi rolls. Dulse can be found in powdered form and can be used like a condiment, or it may be in chunks. Both types of seaweed are high in vitamins and minerals and very low in calories. Check your local health food store or Asian market and try it in this recipe for a real taste of the sea!*

Lentil-Apple Salad

GLUTEN-FREE • DAIRY-FREE
PREP TIME: 10 MINUTES, PLUS 30 MINUTES MARINATING TIME

Apples and lentils are paired together in this energizing salad that will keep you feeling full and satisfied for hours. Apples contain a type of soluble fiber called pectin, which can help lower bad cholesterol and slow down the absorption of your food, especially carbohydrates. They also contain a type of phytochemical that can help prevent spikes in blood sugar. Thyme and tarragon give a French flair to this combination that gets a hint of sweetness from granulated stevia.

1½ teaspoons apple cider vinegar

¼ teaspoon granulated stevia

Pinch salt

Freshly ground black pepper

1 tablespoon extra-virgin olive oil

1½ teaspoons water

1 cup finely diced peeled apple

½ cup finely diced plum tomatoes

1 (14.5-ounce) can lentils, drained and rinsed

1 tablespoon fresh thyme

1 tablespoon fresh tarragon

4 cups mixed salad greens, divided

1. In a large bowl, whisk together the apple cider vinegar, stevia, and salt until the stevia dissolves. Season with pepper.

2. Add the olive oil. Whisk until emulsified.

3. Add the water. Whisk again to loosen.

4. Add the apple and tomatoes. Toss to coat. Let sit for 15 minutes.

5. Add the lentils, thyme, and tarragon. Stir to combine. Let sit for 15 minutes more.

6. Plate 2 cups of salad greens and half of the lentil mixture for each serving.

PER SERVING Calories: 238; Total Fat: 8g; Protein: 12g; Carbohydrates: 33g; Sugars: 7g; Fiber: 7g; Sodium: 10mg

Sunflower-Tuna-Cauliflower Salad

PREP TIME: 20 MINUTES, PLUS 2 HOURS CHILLING TIME

This lighter version of tuna salad uses high-protein nonfat Greek yogurt in place of high-fat mayonnaise. The finished dish has the same mouthfeel and taste without the guilt and excess calories. Tuna is rich in heart-healthy omega-3 fats and the mineral selenium, an important antioxidant that supports thyroid function. Cauliflower adds crunch and 75 percent of your recommended daily amount of vitamin C.

1 (5-ounce) can tuna packed in water, drained

½ cup plain nonfat Greek yogurt

1 teaspoon freshly squeezed lemon juice

1 teaspoon dried dill

1 scallion, chopped

¼ cup sunflower seeds

2 cups fresh chopped cauliflower florets

4 cups mixed salad greens, divided

1. In a medium bowl, mix together the tuna, yogurt, lemon juice, dill, scallion, and sunflower seeds.

2. Add the cauliflower. Toss gently to coat.

3. Cover and refrigerate for at least 2 hours before serving, stirring occasionally.

4. Serve half of the tuna mixture atop 2 cups of salad greens.

PER SERVING Calories: 252; Total Fat: 9g; Protein: 23g; Carbohydrates: 24g; Sugars: 4g; Fiber: 3g; Sodium: 330mg

RECIPE TIP: *Greek yogurt is a nutritional superstar. It has less sugar and nearly twice the protein of regular yogurt—and the added bonus of a creamier texture. The thickness and tangy taste make it a perfect swap for mayo, sour cream, and other fattening dairy products. Try it in cream-based sauces for grains and pastas. It is also great on low-carb pancakes and waffles in place of sugar-filled syrup. Put a few dollops on your pancakes and top with fresh berries. You'll not only add protein, but also cut calories and sugar.*

Sesame Chicken-Almond Slaw

DAIRY-FREE
PREP TIME: 20 MINUTES • COOK TIME: 40 MINUTES

Angel hair cabbage replaces higher-carb pasta and gives this salad a vitamin and mineral boost as well as an Asian flair. Angel hair cabbage is finely shredded cabbage and can be found in the same section of produce where regular coleslaw is sold. High in soluble fiber and vitamins C and K, cabbage is considered to be a very low–glycemic index food. Baked chicken breast gives this light salad a high-protein boost for long-lasting energy and hunger control.

For the dressing

1 tablespoon rice vinegar

1 teaspoon granulated stevia

2 teaspoons extra-virgin olive oil

1 teaspoon water

½ teaspoon sesame oil

¼ teaspoon reduced-sodium soy sauce

Pinch salt

Pinch freshly ground black pepper

For the salad

8 ounces chicken breast, rinsed and drained

4 cups angel hair cabbage

1 cup shredded romaine lettuce

2 tablespoons sliced scallions

2 tablespoons toasted slivered almonds

2 teaspoons toasted sesame seeds

To make the dressing

In a jar with a tight-fitting lid, add the rice vinegar, stevia, olive oil, water, sesame oil, soy sauce, salt, and pepper. Shake well to combine. Set aside.

To make the salad

1. Preheat the oven to 400°F.

2. To a medium baking dish, add the chicken. Place the dish in the preheated oven. Bake for 30 to 40 minutes, or until completely opaque and the temperature registers 165°F on an instant-read thermometer.

3. Remove from the oven. Slice into strips. Set aside.

4. In a large bowl, toss together the cabbage, romaine, scallions, almonds, sesame seeds, and chicken strips. Add the dressing. Toss again to coat the ingredients evenly.

5. Serve immediately.

PER SERVING Calories: 271; Total Fat: 14g; Protein: 30g; Carbohydrates: 8g; Sugars: 4g; Fiber: 4g; Sodium: 156mg

TOSS IT TOGETHER TIP: *Sesame seeds add a nutty taste and a delicate, almost invisible crunch to many Asian dishes. Sprinkle on steamed broccoli drizzled with freshly squeezed lemon juice. Make a healthy dressing by combining sesame seeds and rice vinegar with low-sodium soy sauce and crushed garlic.*

Meatless Taco Salad

QUICK & EASY
PREP TIME: 20 MINUTES

You won't miss the meat in this colorful, zesty vegetarian taco salad. Exploding with fresh flavors and plant-based protein, this salad is quick and easy to assemble. Black olives, extra-virgin olive oil, and avocado add plenty of heart-healthy fats, and you'll get almost half of your day's fiber in one serving. You won't miss the high-fat, high-sodium tortilla chips replaced here by amazingly nutritious and delicious kale chips. This satisfying salad will soon become a favorite for lunch or your next Meatless Monday.

⅓ cup mashed avocado

¼ cup plain nonfat Greek yogurt

2 tablespoons chopped green bell pepper

1 tablespoon chopped scallions

1 tablespoon extra-virgin olive oil

⅛ teaspoon salt

¼ teaspoon chili powder

¼ teaspoon freshly ground black pepper

½ teaspoon ground cumin

3 cups shredded romaine lettuce

8 cherry tomatoes, halved

1 cup canned kidney beans, rinsed and drained

¼ cup sliced black olives

½ cup crushed kale chips, divided

½ cup shredded nonfat Cheddar cheese, divided

1. In a small bowl, stir together the avocado, yogurt, green bell pepper, scallions, olive oil, salt, chili powder, pepper, and cumin. Set aside.

2. In a large bowl, mix the lettuce, tomatoes, kidney beans, and olives.

3. Evenly divide the lettuce mixture between 2 plates.

4. Top each with half of the avocado mixture.

5. Sprinkle each serving with ¼ cup of kale chips and ¼ cup of Cheddar cheese.

6. Enjoy immediately.

PER SERVING Calories: 351; Total Fat: 16g; Protein: 13g; Carbohydrates: 34g; Sugars: 8g; Fiber: 11g; Sodium: 380mg

TOSS IT TOGETHER TIP: *To use up any leftover beans, cheese, olives, or kale chips, make a super-fast and easy "nacho" dish. Layer the kale chips on a plate. Top with beans and cheese. Microwave for 1 to 2 minutes on high until the cheese melts. Add leftover chopped vegetables, olives, and your favorite seasonings. Mix things up—try topping the beans with nonfat mozzarella and fresh basil for an Italian-inspired dish.*

Warm Sweet Potato and Black Bean Salad

DAIRY-FREE
PREP TIME: 5 MINUTES • COOK TIME: 35 MINUTES

This warm salad is perfect for those chilly days when you want a quick and easy hot meal. Wonderfully aromatic rosemary seasons this simple plant-based dish. Sweet potatoes are considered a "superfood" for diabetics. Their low glycemic index makes them a great alternative to white potatoes. Rosemary contains substances that help stimulate the immune system, increase circulation, and improve digestion. A small amount goes a long way to flavor foods.

Extra-virgin olive oil cooking spray

1 large sweet potato, peeled and cubed

1 tablespoon extra-virgin olive oil

1 tablespoon balsamic vinegar

1 teaspoon dried rosemary

¼ teaspoon garlic powder

⅛ teaspoon salt

⅛ teaspoon freshly ground black pepper

1 cup canned black beans, drained and rinsed

2 tablespoons chopped chives

1. Preheat the oven to 450°F.

2. In a small baking dish coated with cooking spray, place the sweet potato cubes. Put the dish in the preheated oven. Bake for 20 to 35 minutes, uncovered, or until tender.

3. In a medium serving bowl, whisk together the olive oil, balsamic vinegar, rosemary, garlic powder, salt, and pepper.

4. Add the black beans and cooked sweet potato to the oil and herb mixture. Toss to coat.

5. Sprinkle with the chives.

6. Serve immediately and enjoy!

PER SERVING Calories: 229; Total Fat: 7g; Protein: 7g; Carbohydrates: 35g; Sugars: 6g; Fiber: 7g; Sodium: 162mg

TOSS IT TOGETHER TIP: *Consider baking several sweet potatoes at once so you can put together a quick meal using leftover beans, meats, or fish. Sweet potato fries are a healthy alternative to frozen French fries. Cut sweet potatoes into strips, drizzle with extra-virgin olive oil, and bake in a 450°F oven for 25 to 30 minutes, depending on their thickness, until crispy. Mashed sweet potatoes with Greek yogurt also make a nutritious and tasty side dish. You can reduce the carbohydrates in your serving of mashed sweet potatoes by mixing in some mashed cauliflower.*

Mozzarella-Tomato Salad

QUICK & EASY

PREP TIME: 10 MINUTES, PLUS 15 MINUTES CHILLING TIME

Simple and satisfying, this Italian-inspired salad is easy and delicious, especially in the summer when tomatoes are at their peak of perfection. Use in-season tomatoes for maximum flavor, and consider growing your own for peak nutrition. Jarred artichoke hearts and roasted red peppers give this salad a gourmet feel, while the beans add additional soluble fiber, slow-digesting carbs, and B vitamins. Fresh basil is best in this salad and can be found year-round in the produce department of most grocery stores.

Fresh mozzarella cheese
    (2 ounces), cut into
    ¾-inch cubes

½ cup cherry
    tomatoes, halved

½ cup cannellini beans,
    drained and rinsed

½ cup artichoke
    hearts, drained

¼ cup jarred roasted
    red peppers

¼ cup chopped scallions

1 tablespoon minced
    fresh basil

1 tablespoon extra-virgin
    olive oil

2 teaspoons balsamic vinegar

⅛ teaspoon salt

4 cups baby spinach, divided

1. In a small bowl, stir together the mozzarella cheese, tomatoes, beans, artichoke hearts, red peppers, and scallions.

2. In another small bowl, whisk the basil, olive oil, balsamic vinegar, and salt until combined.

3. Drizzle the dressing over the cheese and vegetables. Toss to coat. Chill for 15 minutes.

4. Using 2 plates, arrange 2 cups of spinach on each. Top with half of the cheese and vegetable mixture.

5. Serve immediately.

PER SERVING Calories: 207; Total Fat: 5g; Protein: 17g; Carbohydrates: 25g; Sugars: 3g; Fiber: 8g; Sodium: 251mg

TOSS IT TOGETHER TIP: *There are numerous ways to use jarred artichoke hearts and roasted red peppers to boost the flavor and nutrition of other dishes. Stir into egg, chicken, and tuna salads, fold into scrambled eggs or stuff into omelets, arrange over wilted spinach and top with pine nuts, stir into mashed cauliflower or sweet potatoes, fold into pasta and quinoa dishes, or use in soups and sandwiches. The possibilities are limitless!*

Broccoli "Tabouli"

DAIRY-FREE · QUICK & EASY
PREP TIME: 15 MINUTES

Tabouli (also called tabbouleh), a flavorful Mediterranean dish, is traditionally made with a grain like bulgur, quinoa, couscous, or rice, making it high in carbohydrates. This recipe takes a fresh spin on tradition and keeps the flavor while reducing the carbohydrates. The grain is replaced here with grated broccoli and jicama. The vegetables add more nutrients and flavor, but still give the tabouli a traditional texture. Enjoy this dish as a meal-size salad or as a side dish with baked chicken or salmon.

1 broccoli head, trimmed into florets (about 2 cups)

1 large jicama, peeled

1 cup chickpeas, drained and rinsed

2 plum tomatoes, diced

1 medium cucumber, peeled, seeded, and diced

½ cup chopped fresh parsley

½ cup chopped fresh mint

¼ cup chopped red onion

¼ cup freshly squeezed lemon juice

2 tablespoons sunflower seeds

1 tablespoon extra-virgin olive oil

Salt, to season

Freshly ground black pepper, to season

4 cups baby spinach, divided

1. With a grater or food processor, grate the broccoli into grain size pieces until it resembles rice.

2. Repeat with the jicama. You should have about 1 cup.

3. To a large bowl, add the grated broccoli, grated jicama, chickpeas, tomatoes, cucumber, parsley, mint, red onion, lemon juice, sunflower seeds, and olive oil. Toss until well mixed. Season with salt and pepper.

4. Arrange 2 cups of spinach on each of 2 plates.

5. Top each with half of the tabouli mixture.

6. Serve immediately.

PER SERVING Calories: 421; Total Fat: 12g; Protein: 14g; Carbohydrates: 40g; Sugars: 4g; Fiber: 18g; Sodium: 20mg

TOSS IT TOGETHER TIP: *Chickpeas are loaded with fiber, protein, folic acid, and manganese and make a regular healthy food choice for diabetics. Consider roasting leftover chickpeas for a high-protein, easy-to-make healthy snack to eat in place of higher fat and calorie potato chips or crackers. Preheat the oven to 425°F. Place chickpeas on a parchment-lined baking sheet. Mist with extra-virgin olive oil and season to taste. Bake for 25 minutes, stirring at the 15-minute mark.*

Curried Chicken Salad

PREP TIME: 15 MINUTES • COOK TIME: 40 MINUTES

Typically high in fat and sugar, this curry has been through a nutritional makeover. This healthy salad combines protein-rich chicken breast with seeds and nuts, and a dressing made with nonfat Greek yogurt instead of high-fat mayonnaise. The spices used in curries are what make these dishes so nutritious. The composition of curry powder can vary by region. Most commonly, it is a combination of turmeric, fenugreek, coriander, cinnamon, and ginger. In studies, turmeric has been shown to help prevent blood-sugar spikes due, in part, to its anti-inflammatory effects. Curry may also help lower cholesterol levels, making this dish one to regularly include on your menu.

4 ounces chicken breast, rinsed and drained

1 small apple, peeled, cored, and finely chopped

2 tablespoons slivered almonds

1 tablespoon dried cranberries

2 tablespoons chia seeds

¼ cup plain nonfat Greek yogurt

1 tablespoon curry powder

1½ teaspoons Dijon mustard

⅛ teaspoon salt

¼ teaspoon freshly ground black pepper

4 cups chopped romaine lettuce, divided

1. Preheat the oven to 400°F.

2. To a small baking dish, add the chicken. Place the dish in the preheated oven. Bake for 30 to 40 minutes, or until the chicken is completely opaque and registers 165°F on an instant-read thermometer. Remove from the oven. Chop into cubes. Set aside.

3. In a medium bowl, mix together the chicken, apple, almonds, cranberries, and chia seeds.

4. Add the yogurt, curry powder, mustard, salt, and pepper. Toss to coat.

5. On 2 plates, arrange 2 cups of lettuce on each.

6. Top each with one-half of the curried chicken salad.

7. Serve immediately.

PER SERVING Calories: 194; Total Fat: 4g; Protein: 21g; Carbohydrates: 17g; Sugars: 12g; Fiber: 6g; Sodium: 59mg

TOSS IT TOGETHER TIP: *Use leftover chia seeds to thicken soup or gravies, as a "breading" for baked fish or chicken, to thicken meatballs instead of bread crumbs, or mixed into smoothies and hot cereal. Make a healthy pudding by blending 1 cup of unsweetened almond milk or skim milk, ¼ cup of chia seeds, 1 teaspoon of vanilla, and a few drops of liquid stevia. Simply process until smooth and refrigerate for about 10 minutes to thicken.*

Power Salad

DAIRY-FREE • QUICK & EASY
PREP TIME: 15 MINUTES

Powerful is what you will feel after eating this hearty and nutritious power salad. Fueled by the complete protein edamame, with added monounsaturated fats and fiber from creamy avocado, this tasty salad has more than 10 grams of fiber and 20 grams of protein per serving. What makes this salad especially delightful is the simple dressing thickened with chia seeds—a source of heart-healthy omega-3 fats. Use your imagination—try various vegetable combinations to see what suits you best.

For the dressing

1 tablespoon extra-virgin
olive oil
1 tablespoon freshly squeezed
lemon juice
1 tablespoon balsamic vinegar
1 tablespoon chia seeds
1 teaspoon liquid stevia
Pinch salt
Freshly ground black pepper

For the salad

6 cups mixed baby greens
1 cup shelled edamame
1 cup chopped red cabbage
1 cup chopped red bell pepper
1 cup sliced fresh
button mushrooms
½ cup sliced avocado
¼ cup sliced almonds
1 cup pea shoots, divided

To make the dressing

In a small bowl, whisk together the olive oil, lemon juice, balsamic vinegar, chia seeds, and stevia until well combined. Season with salt and pepper.

To make the salad

1. In a large bowl, toss together the mixed greens, edamame, red cabbage, red bell pepper, mushrooms, avocado, and almonds. Drizzle the dressing over the salad. Toss again to coat well.

2. Divide the salad between 2 plates. Top each with ½ cup of pea shoots and serve.

PER SERVING Calories: 435; Total Fat: 24g; Protein: 21g; Carbohydrates: 38g; Sugars: 9g; Fiber: 12g; Sodium: 136mg

Salmon and Baby Greens with Edamame

DAIRY-FREE • QUICK & EASY
PREP TIME: 15 MINUTES • COOK TIME: 10 MINUTES

Omega-3-rich salmon takes center stage here. Salmon is an excellent source of vitamin D, which can be hard to obtain, especially in the winter months. Salmon is also an excellent source of vitamin B_{12}, which supports healthy metabolism and cardiovascular health. Dill, a spice with antibacterial properties, gives this dish a tang, while the carrots add a bright phytochemical finish. The phytochemical antioxidant beta-carotene provides cardiovascular benefits by protecting cells from damage by free radicals. Additionally, beta-carotene is important for night vision. Eat up for good health!

3 teaspoons extra-virgin olive oil, divided

4 cups mixed baby greens, divided

¼ cup edamame

1 teaspoon balsamic vinegar

¼ teaspoon salt

1 (6-ounce) salmon fillet

Extra-virgin olive oil cooking spray

2 tablespoons chopped fresh dill

1. In a large skillet set over medium heat, heat 1½ teaspoons of olive oil.

2. Add 2 cups of baby greens. Cook for 1 minute. Transfer to a medium salad bowl. Repeat with the remaining 1½ teaspoons of olive oil and 2 cups of baby greens.

3. Add the edamame, balsamic vinegar, and salt to the greens. Toss to combine.

4. Place an oven rack about 8 inches from the broiler.

5. Preheat the broiler to high.

6. To a small ovenproof dish, add the salmon. Coat the salmon with cooking spray.

7. Put the dish under the preheated broiler. Broil for 8 to 10 minutes, depending on its thickness, or until the fish is just cooked.

8. Cut the fish in half. Place it on top of the greens.

9. Top with the fresh dill.

10. Serve immediately.

PER SERVING Calories: 384; Total Fat: 23g; Protein: 42g; Carbohydrates: 11g; Sugars: 4g; Fiber: 5g; Sodium: 522mg

Carrot and Cashew Chicken Salad

DAIRY-FREE

PREP TIME: 20 MINUTES • COOK TIME: 25 MINUTES, PLUS 3 MINUTES COOLING TIME

The irresistible and comforting aroma of roasted vegetables entices you to enjoy this protein-packed salad. Baked chicken provides plenty of blood-sugar-stabilizing protein. It's paired here with the terrific taste of roasted carrots and peppers, and finished with crunchy cashews and snap peas. Roasting vegetables actually increases the bioavailability of their nutrients so you get more carotenoids from roasted carrots than you do from steamed or sautéed. Enjoy the aromatic smokiness of this dish and know that you are feeding your body wholesome, nutritious food.

Extra-virgin olive oil
    cooking spray

1 cup carrots rounds

1 red bell pepper, thinly sliced

1½ teaspoons
    granulated stevia

1 tablespoon extra-virgin
    olive oil, divided

¼ teaspoon salt, divided

⅜ teaspoon freshly ground
    black pepper, divided

1 (6-ounce) boneless skinless
    chicken breast, thinly
    sliced across the grain

2 tablespoons
    chopped scallions

1 tablespoon apple
    cider vinegar

1 cup sugar snap peas

4 cups baby spinach

4 tablespoons chopped
    cashews, divided

1. Preheat the oven to 425°F.

2. Coat an 8-by-8-inch baking pan and a rimmed baking sheet with cooking spray.

3. In the prepared baking pan, add the carrots and red bell pepper. Sprinkle with the stevia, 1 teaspoon of olive oil, ⅛ teaspoon of salt, and ⅛ teaspoon of pepper. Toss to coat.

4. Place the pan in the preheated oven. Roast for about 25 minutes, stirring several times, or until tender.

5. About 5 minutes before the vegetables are done, place the sliced chicken in a medium bowl and drizzle with 1 teaspoon of olive oil. Sprinkle with the scallions. Season with the remaining ⅛ teaspoon of salt and ⅛ teaspoon of pepper. Toss to mix. Arrange in a single layer on the prepared baking sheet.

6. Place the sheet in the preheated oven. Roast for 5 to 7 minutes, turning once, or until cooked through.

(continued)

7. Remove the pan with the vegetables and the baking sheet from the oven. Cool for about 3 minutes.

8. In a large salad bowl, mix together the apple cider vinegar, the remaining 1 teaspoon of olive oil, the sugar snap peas, and remaining ⅛ teaspoon of pepper. Let stand 5 minutes to blend the flavors.

9. To finish, add the spinach to the bowl with the dressing and peas. Toss to mix well.

10. Evenly divide between 2 serving plates. Top each with half of the roasted carrots, half of the roasted red bell peppers, and half of the cooked chicken.

11. Sprinkle each with about 2 tablespoons of cashews. Serve warm.

PER SERVING Calories: 373; Total Fat: 15g; Protein: 29g; Carbohydrates: 36g; Sugars: 8g; Fiber: 6g; Sodium: 555mg

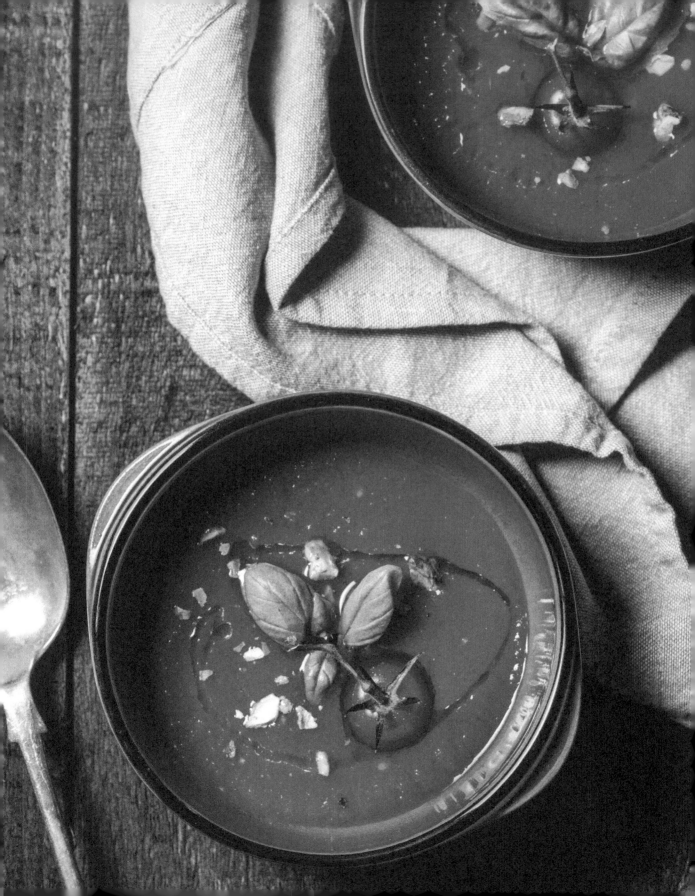

CHAPTER 5

Soups & Stews

Spicy Cioppino

DAIRY-FREE
PREP TIME: 5 MINUTES • COOK TIME: 15 MINUTES

Cioppino (chuh-pee-noh) is a fish stew popular on both U.S. coasts, as well as in Italy where the word "cioppino" originated. Cioppino, similar to bouillabaisse, a French seafood stew, applies the same cooking principle—simmer the catch of the day in a rich broth and enjoy a heart-healthy meal! The seafood assortment can vary and may include mussels, clams, scallops, halibut, or bass. The key is using extremely fresh seafood. Feel free to make substitutions based on the catch of the day at your local grocer.

2 tablespoons extra-virgin olive oil, divided

1 (4-ounce) tilapia fillet, diced

6 medium shrimp, peeled and deveined

1 small sweet onion, sliced

1 shallot, chopped

1 garlic clove, chopped

3 plum tomatoes, diced

2 teaspoons Italian seasoning

2 teaspoons hot paprika

¼ teaspoon salt

¼ teaspoon freshly ground black pepper

1½ cups water

Fresh parsley, for garnish

1. In a large saucepan set over medium-high heat, heat 1 tablespoon of olive oil. Add the tilapia and shrimp. Cook for about 2 minutes, stirring once or twice, until just opaque. Transfer to a plate. Cover with aluminum foil to keep warm. Set aside.

2. Add the remaining 1 tablespoon of olive oil to the pan.

3. Add the onion, shallot, and garlic. Cook for about 2 minutes, stirring frequently, until softened.

4. Add the tomatoes, Italian seasoning, paprika, salt, pepper, and water. Bring to a simmer. Reduce the heat to low. Maintain a simmer and cook for 5 minutes.

5. Add the tilapia and shrimp. Return to a simmer. Cook for about 2 minutes, or until heated through.

6. Garnish with parsley and serve.

PER SERVING Calories: 239; Total Fat: 15g; Protein: 18g; Carbohydrates: 9g; Sugars: 2g; Fiber: 2g; Sodium: 102mg

RECIPE TIP: *Traditional cioppino calls for 1 cup of dry white wine or red wine in the broth, but many people avoid alcohol, even when cooking, for various reasons. The easiest substitute is water, but there are other delicious alternatives you can try. For dry white wine, substitute white wine vinegar, white grape juice with a bit of lemon juice, chicken broth, or vegetable broth. For the red wine, try substituting apple juice, beef broth, or tomato juice.*

Miso Pork and Apple Soup

DAIRY-FREE • QUICK & EASY

PREP TIME: 15 MINUTES • COOK TIME: 10 MINUTES

Pork and apples have been paired together since medieval times when pigs grazed in apple orchards and autumn was the time for prepping meat for the winter months ahead. This modern-day version uses extra-lean pork to limit unhealthy fats, and high-carb noodles are replaced with angel hair coleslaw. The soup gets its sweetness from white miso, a paste made from fermented soybeans. The result is a delicious high-protein soup full of wholesome flavors.

1½ teaspoons extra-virgin olive oil

1 medium sweet onion, chopped

2 garlic cloves, minced

6 ounces extra-lean ground pork

1 tart apple, peeled, cored, and chopped

2 cups water

1 cup reduced-sodium chicken broth

2 cups angel hair coleslaw

1½ tablespoons white miso

1. In a medium saucepan set over medium-high heat, heat the olive oil.

2. Add the onion and garlic. Sauté for about 2 minutes, or until softened.

3. Add the pork. Cook for about 2 minutes, stirring occasionally, until no longer pink.

4. Stir in the apple. Cook for about 2 minutes more, stirring occasionally, until just beginning to soften.

5. Add the water and chicken broth. Bring to a boil.

6. Add the angel hair coleslaw. Cook for 2 minutes until softened.

7. To a small bowl, add the miso.

(continued)

8. Remove ¼ cup of the cooking liquid from the pan and add it to the miso. Whisk until fully dissolved.

9. Stir the miso mixture back into the soup. Remove from the heat.

10. Serve immediately.

PER SERVING Calories: 317; Total Fat: 15g; Protein: 21g; Carbohydrates: 29g; Sugars: 12g; Fiber: 5g; Sodium: 621mg

TOSS IT TOGETHER TIP: *One way to include the health benefits of fermented foods in your diet is to add miso to your cooking staples. Miso paste is a fantastic ingredient you can use in your daily cooking—not just in soup! Due to its health benefits, miso has gone mainstream and can be found in most major grocery stores. There are several types of miso including white, yellow, red, and black. Generally speaking, the darker the color the longer it has been fermented and the stronger the taste. Make a simple miso soup by dissolving 2 tablespoons of the paste in hot water. Miso will keep in the refrigerator for several years.*

Freshened-Up French Onion Soup

PREP TIME: 5 MINUTES • COOK TIME: 30 MINUTES

Traditional French onion soup is basically onions slowly browned combined with a simple beef broth, and topped with a toasted baguette and cheese. It's usually served as a starter. If you think this soup is off-limits, here's some good news! With a few simple swaps, you can enjoy this nourishing and delicious soup without worrying that it has too many carbohydrates. This recipe uses chickpeas to add body. It includes cheese, but lightens it up. You won't even miss the bread!

1 tablespoon extra-virgin olive oil

2 medium onions, sliced

2 cups low-sodium beef broth

1 (8-ounce) can chickpeas, drained and rinsed

½ teaspoon dried thyme

Salt

Freshly ground black pepper

4 slices nonfat Swiss deli-style cheese

1. In a medium soup pot set over medium-low heat, heat the olive oil.

2. Add the onions. Stir to coat them in oil. Cook for about 10 minutes, or until golden brown.

3. Add the beef broth, chickpeas, and thyme. Bring to a simmer.

4. Taste the broth. Season with salt and pepper. Cook for 10 minutes more.

5. Preheat the broiler to high.

6. Ladle the soup into 2 ovenproof soup bowls.

7. Top each with 2 slices of Swiss cheese. Place the bowls on a baking sheet. Carefully transfer the sheet to the preheated oven. Melt the cheese under the broiler for 2 minutes. Alternately, you can melt the cheese in the microwave (in microwave-safe bowls) on high in 30-second intervals until melted.

8. Enjoy immediately.

PER SERVING Calories: 330; Total Fat: 10g; Protein: 27g; Carbohydrates: 37g; Sugars: 11g; Fiber: 10g; Sodium: 402mg

RECIPE TIP: *When you make French onion soup, there are many types of onions to use. Some recipes use red onions, some use white, and some even use dried onion flakes. Select onions that are dry and firm with a shiny outer skin. A fresh onion should have a mild smell. If using a sweet onion, use them within a few days after buying. Many people prefer Vidalia onions for their sweet flavor, but it really comes down to a matter of personal preference.*

Kickin' Chili

DAIRY-FREE
PREP TIME: 10 MINUTES • COOK TIME: 45 MINUTES

There are as many chili recipes as there are cooks, and this simple recipe is just enough for two people. With a nutritional boost from broccoli and the creamy pink texture of pinto beans, you get a satisfying high-protein meal that provides several servings of vegetables in each bowl. Pinto beans—a fiber all-star—contain a whopping 15 grams of fiber in 1 cup, which is more than half your day's requirement. The type of fiber in pinto beans helps stabilize blood-sugar levels while providing steady, slow-burning energy.

1 tablespoon extra-virgin olive oil

½ cup chopped onions

1 garlic clove, minced

1 celery stalk, chopped

½ cup chopped bell peppers, any color

1 cup diced tomatoes, undrained

1 cup frozen broccoli florets

1 (15-ounce) can pinto beans, drained and rinsed

2 cups water

2 teaspoons ground cumin

2 teaspoons chili powder

½ teaspoon cayenne pepper

Salt, to season

Freshly ground black pepper, to season

1. In a large pot set over medium heat, heat the olive oil.

2. Add the onions. Cook for about 5 minutes, or until tender.

3. Add the garlic. Cook for 2 to 3 minutes, or until lightly browned.

4. Add the celery and bell peppers. Cook for 5 minutes, or until the vegetables are soft.

5. Stir in the tomatoes, broccoli, pinto beans, and water.

6. Add the cumin, chili powder, and cayenne pepper. Season with salt and pepper. Stir to combine. Simmer for 30 minutes, stirring frequently.

7. Serve hot and enjoy!

PER SERVING Calories: 300; Total Fat: 7g; Protein: 13g; Carbohydrates: 44g; Sugars: 5g; Fiber: 16g; Sodium: 237mg

TOSS IT TOGETHER TIP: *If you are wondering how to replace meat in some of your meals, consider pinto beans. When beans are combined with a grain, like brown rice, their protein quality equals that of meat or dairy, plus you get the benefit of cholesterol-lowering and blood-sugar-stabilizing fiber. Make an easy sandwich spread or dip by blending pinto beans with sage, oregano, garlic, and black pepper.*

Tasty Tomato Soup

PREP TIME: 10 MINUTES • COOK TIME: 1 HOUR, 25 MINUTES

Prepare your taste buds for this tasty tomato soup made with roasted tomatoes and roasted red peppers. Roasting brings out the natural sweetness in vegetables and intensifies their natural flavors, tantalizing your sense of sight, smell, and taste. Tomatoes are rich in antioxidants, especially lycopene, which can reduce the risk of prostate cancer. Eating tomatoes has also been shown to decrease total cholesterol, LDL "bad" cholesterol, and triglycerides. Once you make this soup, Campbell's will never be the same again!

3 cups chopped tomatoes

1 red bell pepper, cut into chunks

2 tablespoons extra-virgin olive oil, divided

Salt, to season

Freshly ground black pepper, to season

1 medium onion, chopped

1 garlic clove, minced

2 cups low-sodium vegetable broth

1 cup sliced fresh button mushrooms

½ cup fresh chopped basil

1. Preheat the oven to 400°F.

2. On a baking sheet, spread out the tomatoes and red bell pepper.

3. Drizzle with 1 tablespoon of olive oil. Toss to coat. Season with salt and pepper. Place the sheet in the preheated oven. Roast for 45 minutes.

4. In a large stockpot set over medium heat, heat the remaining 1 tablespoon of olive oil.

5. Add the onion. Cook for 2 to 3 minutes, or until tender.

6. Stir in the garlic. Cook for 2 minutes more.

7. Add the vegetable broth, mushrooms, and basil.

8. Stir in the roasted tomatoes and peppers. Reduce the heat to medium-low. Cook for 30 minutes.

(continued)

9. To a blender or food processor, carefully transfer the soup in batches, blending until smooth. Return the processed soup to the pot. Simmer for 5 minutes.

10. Serve warm and enjoy!

PER SERVING Calories: 286; Total Fat: 14g; Protein: 8g; Carbohydrates: 31g; Sugars: 16g; Fiber: 9g; Sodium: 493mg

TOSS IT TOGETHER TIP: *You can use olive oil cooking spray instead of oil when roasting vegetables. Simply spray the vegetables on both sides and sprinkle with your desired seasonings, such as rosemary, basil, parsley, marjoram, salt, and pepper. You can roast just about any vegetable—carrots, beets, peppers, garlic, eggplant, asparagus, Brussels sprouts, summer squash, and onions. Roasting can turn most self-proclaimed vegetable haters into vegetable lovers!*

Italian Meatball-Zucchini "Noodle" Soup

DAIRY-FREE
PREP TIME: 15 MINUTES • COOK TIME: 30 MINUTES

Enjoying your favorite foods is easy to do, even when watching your total carbohydrate intake. Italian meatball soup typically contains pasta and meatballs made with bread crumbs. In this recipe, low-calorie zucchini "noodles" replace the pasta, and chia seeds bind the meatballs, along with egg as a bread crumb replacement. If you don't have a spiral slicer, slice the zucchini into thin strips with a julienne peeler, or substitute angel hair coleslaw.

1 large egg, lightly beaten

1 tablespoon chia seeds

¼ cup minced fresh parsley

Salt, to season

Freshly ground black pepper, to season

¼ pound (93 percent) lean ground beef

Extra-virgin olive oil cooking spray

1 medium carrot, thinly sliced

1 celery stalk, chopped

1 small onion, chopped

1 tablespoon tomato paste

2 teaspoons Italian seasoning

1 teaspoon dried oregano

2 cups diced tomatoes

2 cups low-sodium beef broth

1 medium zucchini, spiral-sliced

1. In a small bowl, blend together the egg, chia seeds, and parsley. Season with salt and pepper.

2. Crumble the beef into the bowl. Mix well. Shape into 1-inch balls.

3. In a large saucepan set over medium heat, brown the meatballs for about 5 minutes per side, turning frequently. Drain and set aside.

4. Lightly spray a large soup pot with cooking spray.

5. Add the carrot, celery, and onion. Cook for 4 to 5 minutes, stirring occasionally, or until the vegetables begin to brown. Push the vegetables to one side of the pot.

6. Add the tomato paste to the side of the pot without the vegetables. Cook for 1 to 2 minutes, or until the paste begins to caramelize.

7. Add the Italian seasoning and oregano. Mix well.

(continued)

8. Stir in the tomatoes and beef broth. Mix the ingredients together. Bring to a simmer.

9. Add the meatballs and zucchini "noodles." Simmer for 10 to 12 minutes more.

10. Season the soup with salt and pepper.

11. Serve hot.

PER SERVING Calories: 267; Total Fat: 8g; Protein: 24g; Carbohydrates: 25g; Sugars: 12g; Fiber: 10g; Sodium: 272mg

RECIPE TIP: *Vegetable spiralizers and julienne peelers are kitchen gadgets you may want to add to your stock of essential tools— especially for low-carbohydrate cooking. Peelers can be found for under ten dollars. They can be used to turn carrots, zucchini, and yellow squash into huge bowls of pasta-like veggies that you won't feel guilty about eating! There's nothing more fun than a new kitchen gadget, especially one that won't gather dust.*

Asparagus Soup

DAIRY-FREE • QUICK & EASY
PREP TIME: 5 MINUTES • COOK TIME: 10 MINUTES

This highly prized vegetable arrives with spring when its shoots break through the soil and reach their harvest length of six to eight inches. Generally, the growing season for asparagus is April through May, which is a perfect time to make this light, nourishing soup. Asparagus is another top vegetable choice for blood-sugar control due to its high content of a unique type of fiber called inulin. Enjoy this delectable vegetable paired with high-protein, high-fiber cannellini beans in this easy-to-make soup.

1 pound asparagus, woody ends removed, sliced into 1-inch pieces

1 (8-ounce) can cannellini beans, drained and rinsed

2 cups reduced-sodium vegetable broth

1 medium shallot, thinly sliced

1 garlic clove, thinly sliced

½ teaspoon dried thyme

½ teaspoon dried marjoram leaves

⅛ teaspoon salt

Freshly ground black pepper, to season

1. In a large saucepan set over high heat, stir together the asparagus, cannellini beans, vegetable broth, shallot, garlic, thyme, marjoram, and salt. Bring to a boil. Reduce the heat to medium-low. Cover and simmer for about 5 minutes, or until the asparagus is tender.

2. In a large blender or food processor, purée the soup until smooth, scraping down the sides, if necessary. Season with pepper.

3. Serve immediately and enjoy!

PER SERVING Calories: 150; Total Fat: 1g; Protein: 9g; Carbohydrates: 26g; Sugars: 6g; Fiber: 8g; Sodium: 182mg

TOSS IT TOGETHER TIP: *Thin asparagus doesn't require peeling. Asparagus with thick stems should be peeled, however, because the stems are usually tough and stringy. Remove the tough outer skin from the bottom portion of the stem (not the tips) with a vegetable peeler, and rinse under cold water to remove any soil residue. Chopped asparagus makes a great addition to omelets and can be added, cold, to your favorite salad.*

Seafood Stew

DAIRY-FREE · QUICK & EASY
PREP TIME: 10 MINUTES · COOK TIME: 10 MINUTES

This seafood stew combines fresh fish with green beans and peas for a hearty dish rich in flavor as well as color. We don't usually think of peas as a nutritional standout, but we should. Peas get that sweet taste and texture from their sugar and starch content, but they are actually an excellent support for blood-sugar regulation due to their substantial amounts of protein and fiber. Bursting with nutrition from heart-healthy fish and phytochemical-rich vegetables, this quick and easy stew is sure to become a mealtime favorite.

2 teaspoons extra-virgin olive oil

1 medium onion, chopped

1 small red bell pepper, chopped

1 garlic clove, chopped

1 teaspoon dried sage

½ teaspoon fennel seed

¼ teaspoon salt

¼ teaspoon freshly ground black pepper

Pinch saffron threads

1 cup no-salt-added diced tomatoes, with juice

¼ cup low-sodium chicken broth

⅔ cup frozen peas

1 cup green beans, cut into 1-inch pieces

4 ounces bay scallops, tough muscle removed

4 ounces small shrimp, peeled and deveined

1. In a large saucepan set over medium heat, heat the olive oil.

2. Add onion and red bell pepper. Cook for 3 minutes, stirring constantly.

3. Add the garlic, sage, fennel seed, salt, pepper, and saffron. Cook for 20 seconds.

4. Stir in the tomatoes, chicken broth, peas, and green beans. Bring to a simmer. Cover and reduce the heat to low. Simmer for 2 minutes. Increase the heat to medium.

5. Stir in the scallops. Cook for 2 minutes, stirring occasionally.

6. Add the shrimp. Cook for 2 minutes more, stirring occasionally.

7. Serve hot and enjoy!

PER SERVING Calories: 266; Total Fat: 6g; Protein: 27g; Carbohydrates: 26g; Sugars: 11g; Fiber: 6g; Sodium: 285mg

TOSS IT TOGETHER TIP: *Saffron, the dried, aromatic stigma from the* Crocus sativus *family, has always been considered precious. Saffron adds flavor and golden color to a variety of Middle Eastern, African, and European foods and a little goes a long way. Saffron is especially good in paella and risottos. Make a marinade for fish by adding saffron threads, garlic, and thyme to vinegar. Find it in the spice section of most supermarkets. It will keep in an airtight container for several years.*

Chock-Full-of-Vegetables Chicken Soup

DAIRY-FREE • QUICK & EASY
PREP TIME: 5 MINUTES • COOK TIME: 15 MINUTES

Chock full of vegetables aptly describes this loaded chicken soup, which will hit the spot on a cold winter day. High in protein and fiber, you won't miss the noodles as you fill up on zucchini, mushrooms, tomatoes, spinach, and carrots. Marjoram adds a mild, sweet, oregano-like flavor, bringing out the flavor of the vegetables. The chicken tenders keep the fat content low. Enjoy this soup with a side of kale chips as a healthy alternative to saltines.

1 tablespoon extra virgin
   olive oil

8 ounces chicken tenders, cut
   into bite-size chunks

1 small zucchini, finely diced

1 cup sliced fresh
   button mushrooms

2 medium carrots,
   thinly sliced

2 celery stalks, thinly sliced

1 large shallot, finely chopped

1 garlic clove, minced

1 tablespoon dried parsley

1 teaspoon dried marjoram

⅛ teaspoon salt

2 plum tomatoes, chopped

2 cups reduced-sodium
   chicken broth

1½ cups packed baby spinach

1. In a large saucepan set over medium high heat, heat olive oil.

2. Add the chicken. Cook for 3 to 4 minutes, stirring occasionally, or until browned. Transfer to a plate. Set aside.

3. To the saucepan, add the zucchini, mushrooms, carrots, celery, shallot, garlic, parsley, marjoram, and salt. Cook for 2 to 3 minutes, stirring frequently, until the vegetables are slightly softened.

4. Add the tomatoes and chicken broth. Increase the heat to high. Bring to a boil, stirring occasionally. Reduce the heat to low. Simmer for 5 minutes, or until the vegetables are tender.

5. Stir in the spinach, cooked chicken, and any accumulated juices on the plate. Cook for about 2 minutes, stirring, until the chicken is heated through.

6. Serve hot and enjoy!

PER SERVING Calories: 309; Total Fat: 8g; Protein: 35g; Carbohydrates: 24g; Sugars: 7g; Fiber: 10g; Sodium: 558mg

Lentil Stew

DAIRY-FREE

PREP TIME: 10 MINUTES • COOK TIME: 30 MINUTES

This hearty stew is loaded with heart-healthy fiber and plant-based protein from the small but mighty lentil. Lentils are a superstar among beans and, compared to other beans, are quick and easy to prepare. They readily absorb flavors from other foods and seasonings and can be used in a variety of dishes. Lentils also give you slow-burning energy that helps balance blood-sugar levels. Rich in protein, fiber, and iron, this delicious and satisfying stew can be served for breakfast, lunch, or dinner.

½ cup dry lentils, picked through, debris removed, rinsed and drained

2½ cups water

1 bay leaf

2 teaspoons dried tarragon

2 teaspoons dried thyme

2 garlic cloves, minced

2 medium carrots, chopped

2 medium tomatoes, diced

1 celery stalk, chopped

1 tablespoon extra-virgin olive oil

1 medium onion, diced

1 cup frozen spinach

Salt, to season

Freshly ground black pepper, to season

1. In a soup pot set over high heat, stir together the lentils, water, bay leaf, tarragon, thyme, and garlic.

2. Add the carrots, tomatoes, and celery. Cover. Bring to a boil. Reduce the heat to low and stir the soup. Simmer for 15 to 20 minutes, covered, or until the lentils are tender.

3. While the vegetables simmer, place a skillet over medium heat. Add the olive oil and onion. Sauté for about 10 minutes, or until browned. Remove the skillet from the heat.

4. When the lentils are tender, remove and discard the bay leaf. Add the cooked onion and the spinach to the soup. Heat for 5 to 10 minutes more, or until the spinach is cooked.

5. Season with salt and pepper.

6. Enjoy immediately.

PER SERVING Calories: 258; Total Fat: 8g; Protein: 16g; Carbohydrates: 45g; Sugars: 14g; Fiber: 18g; Sodium: 107mg

TOSS IT TOGETHER TIP: *Cook a big pot of lentils to eat throughout the week. Add them to omelets and salads, or use in place of starchy carbs as a nutritious side to baked fish or poultry. Lentils don't need to be soaked before cooking, but they should be washed and picked through to remove any debris. Sold whole or split, varieties include green, brown, black, yellow, red, and orange.*

Pumpkin and Black Bean Soup

DAIRY-FREE

PREP TIME: 15 MINUTES • COOK TIME: 35 MINUTES

There are many more uses for pumpkin than just making a sugar-filled pie. Surprisingly, soup is one of them. The pumpkin's bright orange color is a dead giveaway that this vegetable is loaded with the antioxidant beta-carotene and vitamin A. Pumpkin is very low in calories, high in fiber, and high in blood-pressure-regulating potassium. Combined with high-fiber, high-protein black beans, this satisfying soup is easy to make and yummy to eat.

2 teaspoons extra virgin olive oil

1 small onion, finely chopped

1 small red bell pepper, chopped

1 garlic clove, minced

1 teaspoon ground cumin

1 cup low-sodium vegetable broth

1 cup diced tomatoes, with juice

1 cup canned black beans, drained and rinsed

1 (8-ounce) can solid-pack pumpkin

1 cup almond milk, or soy milk

½ cup frozen spinach

Salt, to season

Freshly ground black pepper, to season

Chopped fresh chives, for garnish

1. In a medium pot set over medium heat, heat the olive oil.

2. Stir in the onion and bell pepper. Cook for about 5 minutes, stirring, until the onion softens and turns translucent.

3. Mix in the garlic and cumin. Cook, stirring, for 2 minutes more.

4. Add the vegetable broth, tomatoes, black beans, pumpkin, almond milk, and spinach. Stir to combine.

5. Season with salt and pepper.

6. Bring the soup to a gentle boil. Reduce the heat to low. Simmer, covered, for 25 minutes.

7. Garnish each bowl of soup with chives and enjoy!

PER SERVING Calories: 266; Total Fat: 7g; Protein: 13g; Carbohydrates: 38g; Sugars: 10g; Fiber: 18g; Sodium: 332mg

TOSS IT TOGETHER TIP: *Canned pumpkin is a great kitchen staple to add to all sorts of dishes—from savory to sweet. Add ½ cup to your morning oats for additional creaminess, add it to smoothies and pancakes, and mix it into risottos. Pumpkin also makes a great sauce for vegetable noodles: sauté onion and garlic, add pumpkin purée, vegetable broth, and sage or rosemary.*

African Peanut Stew

DAIRY-FREE
PREP TIME: 10 MINUTES • COOK TIME: 35 MINUTES

This nutritious stew is great for peanut butter lovers. It's also rich and hearty and super easy to make. Traditional African peanut stew uses chicken and collards, but this vegetarian version maintains the protein in a plant-based form and uses milder-tasting kale for the greens. The vegetables infuse the stew with fiber and antioxidants and an indulgent taste. Use natural, unsalted peanut butter for the most nutrition and to avoid added sugars and unhealthy hydrogenated fats.

3 cups low-sodium
   vegetable broth

1 small onion, chopped

1 small red bell
   pepper, chopped

1 medium carrot, chopped

1 tablespoon minced
   fresh ginger

2 garlic cloves, minced

¼ teaspoon salt, plus more
   to season

½ cup unsalted natural
   peanut butter

2 tablespoons tomato paste

1 bunch kale, thoroughly
   washed, deveined, and
   chopped (about 2½ cups)

Freshly ground black pepper,
   to season

2 scallions, chopped

1. In a medium pot set over medium-low heat, bring the vegetable broth to a boil.

2. Add the onion, bell pepper, carrot, ginger, garlic, and salt. Cook for 20 minutes.

3. In a medium, heat-safe mixing bowl, stir together the peanut butter and tomato paste.

4. Transfer 1 cup of the hot vegetable broth to the bowl. Whisk until smooth. Pour the peanut butter mixture back into the soup. Mix well to combine.

5. Stir in the kale. Season with salt and pepper. Simmer for about 15 minutes more, stirring frequently.

6. Top with the scallions and enjoy!

PER SERVING Calories: 497; Total Fat: 33g; Protein: 22g; Carbohydrates: 38g; Sugars: 10g; Fiber: 13g; Sodium: 557mg

Eggplant Stew

DAIRY-FREE

PREP TIME: 5 MINUTES • COOK TIME: 1 HOUR, 10 MINUTES

This terrific stew is loaded with succulent Mediterranean vegetables and is reminiscent of ratatouille. The addition of black-eyed peas adds protein and blood-sugar-stabilizing fiber. Eggplant is rich in antioxidant compounds, which have been shown to protect both the brain and the heart. Tasty and nutritious, the key to this flavorful dish is the magical melding of flavors that happens during the simmering time. This fragrant stew can be served hot or cold, as an appetizer, main dish, or side dish.

1 tablespoon extra-virgin olive oil

1 small Vidalia onion, chopped

2 garlic cloves, chopped

1 small red bell pepper, chopped

1 small eggplant, chopped

1 cup black-eyed peas, fresh or frozen

1 medium tomato, diced with juice

2 teaspoons dried basil

2 teaspoons dried oregano

⅛ teaspoon salt

3 cups water

1 tablespoon red wine vinegar

1. To a large saucepan set over medium heat, and the olive oil and onion. Sauté for about 5 minutes.

2. Add the garlic and bell pepper. Sauté for 5 minutes more, or until the vegetables just begin to soften.

3. Add the eggplant, black-eyed peas, tomato, basil, oregano, salt, and water. Increase the heat to high. Bring to a boil. Reduce the heat to medium-low. Simmer for about 1 hour, or until the eggplant is completely cooked and tender.

4. Stir in the red wine vinegar. Cook for 2 minutes more.

5. Serve immediately and enjoy!

PER SERVING Calories: 300; Total Fat: 7g; Protein: 13g; Carbohydrates: 45g; Sugars: 14g; Fiber: 11g; Sodium: 29mg

RECIPE TIP: *Choose eggplants that are firm and heavy for their size. The skin should be smooth and shiny, and the color should be vivid. Although they look hardy, eggplants are actually very perishable and should be refrigerated. When making this stew, if too much water evaporates as you are cooking, add more. If the stew looks too watery after the eggplant has cooked, continue cooking until it thickens.*

Green Ginger Soup

DAIRY-FREE

PREP TIME: 10 MINUTES • COOK TIME: 30 MINUTES

This warming soup is loaded with green vegetables puréed to a creamy, smooth finish. The frozen lima beans, green beans, and uncooked rice make this dish easy to prep so you have a nutritious meal in minutes. Pungent, spicy, fresh ginger adds zest and a host of vitamins, minerals, and antioxidants, including calcium, iron, potassium, and vitamins C and E. Used medicinally for several centuries, ginger aids digestion, boosts the immune system, has anticarcinogenic properties, and acts as a powerful anti-inflammatory.

½ cup chopped onion

½ cup peeled, chopped fennel

1 small zucchini, chopped

½ cup frozen lima beans

¼ cup uncooked brown rice

1 bay leaf

1 teaspoon dried basil

⅛ teaspoon freshly ground black pepper

2 cups water

1 cup frozen green beans

¼ cup fresh parsley, chopped

1 (3-inch) piece fresh ginger, peeled, grated, and pressed through a strainer to extract the juice (about 2 to 3 tablespoons)

Salt, to season

2 tablespoons chopped fresh chives

1. In a large pot set over medium-high heat, stir together the onion, fennel, zucchini, lima beans, rice, bay leaf, basil, pepper, and water. Bring to a boil. Reduce the heat to low. Simmer for 15 minutes.

2. Add the green beans. Simmer for about 5 minutes, uncovered, until tender.

3. Stir in the parsley.

4. Remove and discard the bay leaf.

5. In a blender or food processor, purée the soup in batches until smooth, adding water if necessary to thin.

6. Blend in the ginger juice.

7. Season with salt. Garnish with the chives.

8. Serve hot and enjoy immediately!

PER SERVING Calories: 178; Total Fat: 1g; Protein: 6g; Carbohydrates: 35g; Sugars: 3g; Fiber: 6g; Sodium: 140mg

White Bean Soup

DAIRY-FREE
PREP TIME: 15 MINUTES • COOK TIME: 20 MINUTES

Jarred roasted red peppers add a flavor boost to this simple, nutritious white bean soup. Like other beans, white beans are high in minerals, fiber, and protein and provide slow-burning energy that stabilizes blood sugar. Spinach adds calcium and a soluble fiber boost, while rosemary gives the soup a wonderful smell and pungent flavor. Rosemary contains substances that stimulate the immune system, increase circulation, and improve digestion.

1 teaspoon extra virgin
    olive oil

⅓ cup chopped yellow onion

1 garlic clove, minced

1 teaspoon dried rosemary

½ cup sliced
    fresh mushrooms

½ cup jarred roasted red
    peppers, chopped

1 teaspoon freshly squeezed
    lemon juice

1 teaspoon white wine vinegar

1 cup water

1 (15-ounce) can white beans,
    drained and rinsed

½ cup diced tomatoes,
    with juice

1½ cups fresh spinach

1. In a large pot set over medium heat, heat the olive oil.

2. Add the onion and garlic. Sauté for about 5 minutes, or until tender.

3. Add the rosemary, mushrooms, red peppers, lemon juice, white wine vinegar, and water. Cook for 5 minutes more, or until the mushrooms are soft.

4. Stir in the white beans, tomatoes, and spinach. Cook for 10 minutes more, or until the spinach is wilted.

5. Serve immediately and enjoy!

PER SERVING Calories: 277; Total Fat: 4g; Protein: 16g; Carbohydrates: 44g; Sugars: 4g; Fiber: 12g; Sodium: 380mg

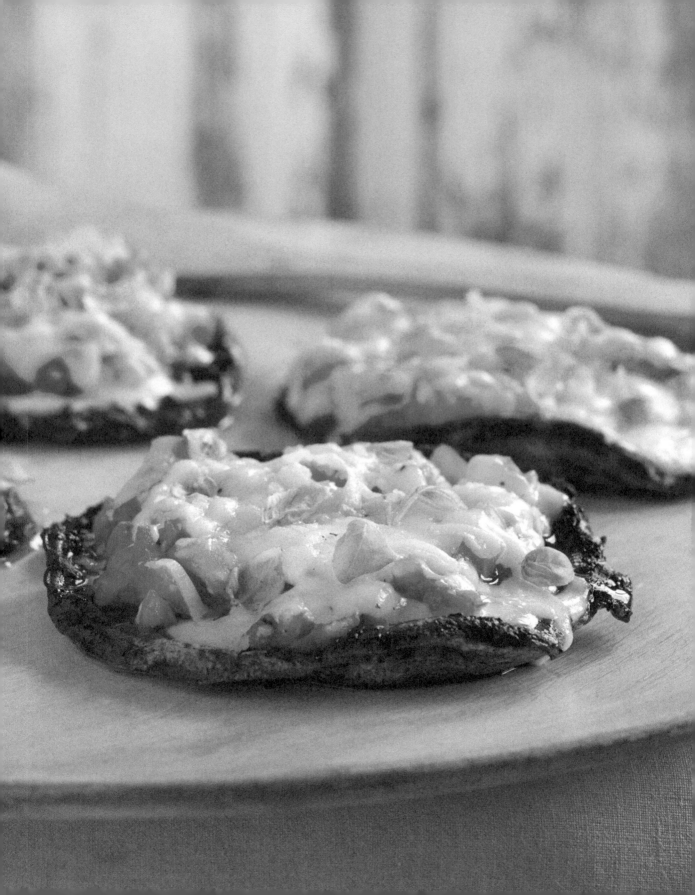

CHAPTER 6

Comfort Classics

Mock Mac and Cheese

PREP TIME: 5 MINUTES • COOK TIME: 45 MINUTES

With this creative recipe, you get all the creamy, cheesy goodness of traditional mac and cheese without the high-starch content of macaroni. Cauliflower florets make a fantastic replacement for pasta—and, admit it, when you eat mac and cheese, you savor the creamy richness of the cheese, not the pasta! To make this even healthier, the cheese is thickened with low-carb coconut flour instead of wheat flour. Nutritional yeast boosts the B vitamins and gives it even more cheesy flavor. Topped with toasted wheat germ instead of high-carb bread crumbs for that added crunch, this dish is sure to please.

Extra-virgin olive oil cooking spray

2 cups cauliflower florets

2 teaspoons extra-virgin olive oil

1 tablespoon coconut flour

½ cup nonfat milk

1 garlic clove, minced

½ cup shredded nonfat Cheddar cheese

¼ cup nutritional yeast

Pinch cayenne pepper

1 large egg yolk

4 tablespoons toasted wheat germ, divided

1. Preheat the oven to 350°F.

2. Spray 2 (8-ounce) ramekins with cooking spray. Set aside.

3. Bring a medium pot of salted water to a boil over high heat.

4. Add the cauliflower. Boil for 5 minutes, or until just tender. Drain, reserving ¼ cup of the cooking liquid. Set aside.

5. In the same pot set over medium heat, heat the olive oil.

6. Whisk in the coconut flour. Cook for 1 minute, stirring constantly.

7. Whisk in the milk, garlic, and reserved cooking liquid. Cook for 7 to 10 minutes, or until thickened, whisking constantly. Remove from the heat.

8. Stir in the Cheddar cheese, yeast, cayenne pepper, and egg yolk. Continue stirring until the cheese melts.

9. Fold in the cauliflower.

10. Evenly divide the cauliflower mixture between the ramekins.

11. Sprinkle each serving with about 2 tablespoons of the wheat germ. Spray the wheat germ with cooking spray.

12. Place the ramekins on a baking sheet. Carefully transfer the sheet to the preheated oven. Bake for 30 minutes, or until the casseroles are hot and bubbly and the wheat germ is crisp and brown.

PER SERVING Calories: 338; Total Fat: 10g; Protein: 31g; Carbohydrates: 39g; Sugars: 7g; Fiber: 11g; Sodium: 354mg

TOSS IT TOGETHER TIP: *Toasted wheat germ is an excellent source of vitamin E, B vitamins, omega-3 fats, fiber, protein, and essential minerals and should be part of every cook's list of kitchen staples. Use it to make a healthy "breading," add it to cooked hot cereal or pancake batter, mix it into smoothies, sprinkle it on yogurt or salads, and top cooked vegetables with it. Wheat germ has a nutty flavor and crunch consistency and should be refrigerated to keep it fresh.*

Spaghetti Squash with Marinara

PREP TIME: 15 MINUTES • COOK TIME: 45 MINUTES

No, spaghetti squash isn't *exactly* like spaghetti pasta—it's more tender than it is chewy, and has a lighter and cleaner flavor, somewhere between butternut squash and zucchini—but it does make a darn good substitute if you're watching your carbs. Plus, using it in place of pasta adds at least two vegetable servings to your day. Who can argue with that? Another perk when cooking for two is that this vegetable is perfectly portioned. Just cook, cut in half, and scoop out the strands from each half, per person. Low in calories and high in vitamins, minerals, and fiber, spaghetti squash is a great choice for any weight-management plan.

For the "spaghetti"

1 medium spaghetti squash, halved lengthwise, seeds removed

For the marinara

1 teaspoon extra-virgin olive oil

1 small onion, chopped

1 portobello mushroom cap, coarsely chopped

1 garlic clove, minced

1 (8-ounce) can no-salt-added diced tomatoes

1 teaspoon Italian seasoning

½ cup shredded nonfat mozzarella cheese, divided

Salt, to season

Freshly ground black pepper, to season

To make the "spaghetti"

1. Preheat the oven to 350°F.

2. In a large baking dish, place the squash halves cut-side down. With a fork, prick the skin all over. Place the dish into the preheated oven. Bake for 30 to 40 minutes, or until tender.

To make the marinara

1. In a medium skillet set over medium-high heat, heat the olive oil.

2. Add the onion, mushroom, and garlic. Sauté for about 5 minutes, or until tender.

3. Stir in the tomatoes and Italian seasoning. Bring to a boil. Reduce the heat to low. Simmer for about 5 minutes, uncovered, stirring frequently, or until it is the desired consistency.

To serve

1. Using a fork, carefully rake the stringy pulp from the squash, separating into spaghetti-like strands, and fluff. Divide the strands between 2 plates.

2. Top each plate with half of the marinara.

3. Sprinkle each with ¼ cup of mozzarella cheese. Season with salt and pepper.

4. Enjoy immediately!

PER SERVING Calories: 233; Total Fat: 2g; Protein: 14g; Carbohydrates: 41g; Sugars: 16g; Fiber: 8g; Sodium: 389mg

RECIPE TIP: *Spaghetti squash and other types of winter squash, like acorn and butternut, can be cooked in the microwave if you're short on time. Simply pierce the squash several times on all sides with a small, sharp knife. Microwave in a large dish with about ¼ cup of water on high for 3 to 4 minutes. Carefully turn the squash and microwave for 3 to 4 minutes more, or until tender.*

Portobello Mushroom Pizzas

PREP TIME: 5 MINUTES • COOK TIME: 25 MINUTES

Pizza is often greasy and loaded with saturated fats and calories from the cheese and processed meats. Consuming saturated fats and excess calories on a regular basis puts you at an increased risk for heart disease and obesity. But there's good news! Portobello mushroom caps make a creative, chewy, delicious substitute for unhealthy pizza crusts—and they come pre-portioned! Very low in calories, portobello mushrooms are a good source of fiber and B vitamins, and are high in the mineral selenium, an important antioxidant that supports immune function. Experiment with toppings and enjoy this quick and easy healthy pizza for a quick lunch or light dinner.

2 large portobello
  mushroom caps

1 tablespoon extra-virgin
  olive oil

1 teaspoon dried oregano

½ teaspoon red pepper flakes

Salt, to season

Freshly ground black pepper,
  to season

1 cup shredded nonfat
  mozzarella cheese, divided

1 medium tomato,
  sliced, divided

3 teaspoons sliced black
  olives, divided

4 tablespoons chopped fresh
  basil, divided

1. Preheat the oven to 375°F.

2. On a baking sheet, place the mushrooms. Put the sheet in the preheated oven. Bake for 5 minutes. Remove from the oven.

3. Drizzle the mushrooms with the olive oil.

4. Sprinkle with the oregano and red pepper flakes. Season with salt and pepper.

5. Spread ½ cup of mozzarella cheese in each mushroom cap.

6. Top each with half of the tomato slices, 1½ teaspoons of the black olives, and about 2 tablespoons of basil.

7. Top each with ¼ cup of the remaining mozzarella cheese.

8. Return to the oven. Bake for 20 minutes, or until the cheese melts and is golden.

PER SERVING Calories: 152; Total Fat: 8g; Protein: 11g; Carbohydrates: 9g; Sugars: 4g; Fiber: 2g; Sodium: 348mg

TOSS IT TOGETHER TIP: *There are lots of ways to use leftover olives and reap the benefits of their heart-healthy monounsaturated fats. Wake up a green salad with olives and avocado slices; add sliced olives to scrambled eggs, omelets, and frittatas; stir chopped olives into tuna, chicken, or seafood salad, or hot quinoa or brown rice.*

Eggplant Lasagna

PREP TIME: 15 MINUTES • COOK TIME: 50 MINUTES

Traditional lasagna is heavy in calories, as well as fat, cholesterol, and carbs—qualities that don't mesh with a healthy eating plan. This recipe keeps the pasta, but lightens the dish by using less of it, along with nonfat cheeses and more vegetables to ensure a hearty and satisfying result. Choose whole-wheat lasagna noodles to increase the fiber and protein, and avoid refined carbs. Fresh tomatoes replace spaghetti sauce to give the dish a fresher flavor. Best of all, this recipe is just for two so you don't have a huge pan of leftover lasagna to manage.

Extra-virgin olive oil
    cooking spray

2 eggplant slices, ¼-inch
    thick, cut lengthwise from
    a long eggplant

1 large egg white

½ cup nonfat ricotta cheese

1 tablespoon chopped
    fresh basil

1 garlic clove, minced

¼ teaspoon salt

½ cup chopped
    fresh mushrooms

½ cup frozen spinach

¼ cup chopped red
    bell pepper

1 cup diced tomatoes,
    with juice

1 tablespoon Italian seasoning

2 sheets whole-wheat oven-
    ready lasagna noodles

¼ cup nonfat shredded
    mozzarella cheese

1. Preheat the oven to 425°F.

2. Spray both sides of the eggplant slices with cooking spray. Place on a baking sheet and into the preheated oven. Bake for 10 minutes. Carefully turn the slices over. Bake for 10 minutes more, or until browned and softened.

3. In a medium bowl, blend together the egg white, ricotta cheese, basil, garlic, and salt. Mix well. Set aside.

4. Spray a nonstick skillet with cooking spray. Place it over medium-high heat.

5. Add the mushrooms, spinach, and bell pepper. Cook for about 4 minutes, stirring occasionally, or until softened.

6. Add the vegetables to the ricotta mixture. Stir to combine. Set aside.

7. In a small bowl, stir together the tomatoes and Italian seasoning. Set aside.

8. Spray a large loaf pan with cooking spray.

(continued)

9. Pour ¼ cup of the seasoned tomatoes evenly over the bottom of the pan. Top with 1 lasagna sheet. Spread half of the ricotta-vegetable mixture on top. Cover with another ¼ cup of the tomatoes. Top with 1 eggplant slice.

10. Repeat another layer with ¼ cup of tomatoes, 1 lasagna sheet, the remaining half of the ricotta-vegetable mixture, the remaining ¼ cup of tomatoes, and the remaining 1 eggplant slice.

11. Spread the mozzarella cheese over the top.

12. Place the pan in the preheated oven. Bake for 20 to 25 minutes, or until the cheese starts to brown.

13. Serve and enjoy!

PER SERVING Calories: 215; Total Fat: 3g; Protein: 16g; Carbohydrates: 31g; Sugars: 7g; Fiber: 7g; Sodium: 326mg

TOSS IT TOGETHER TIP: *If you have leftover eggplant, cube it or slice it, blanch it and freeze it so you have some on hand for other recipes. You can also sauté it with scallions, green peppers, and fresh tomatoes, drizzle with extra-virgin olive oil, add basil, and enjoy as a quick side dish. Eggplant can also be breaded (try wheat germ, flaxseed meal, or almond meal) and grilled or fried, and topped with hummus or other favorite toppings.*

Stuffed Sweet Potato Skins

QUICK & EASY
PREP TIME: 10 MINUTES • COOK TIME: 20 MINUTES

This recipe makes a super-fast, healthy meal and is stuffed with nutrition. Edamame are a complete source of high-quality protein and lower in carbohydrates than beans, making them a perfect choice to pair with a baked sweet potato. High-fat sour cream is replaced by nonfat Greek yogurt, which has the same rich consistency. A mix of chili powder and cumin gives this dish its Mexican flavor. Avocado slices as a garnish add a serving of heart-healthy fats and some creamy goodness.

1 medium sweet potato

¼ cup plain nonfat
 Greek yogurt

½ teaspoon chili powder

½ teaspoon paprika

½ teaspoon ground cumin

1 teaspoon extra-virgin
 olive oil

½ cup chopped red
 bell pepper

¼ cup chopped red onion

Pinch salt

Freshly ground black pepper,
 to season

½ cup fresh, or frozen,
 shelled edamame

4 tablespoons shredded
 nonfat Cheddar
 cheese, divided

4 tablespoons salsa, divided

½ small avocado, sliced

Fresh cilantro, for garnish

1. Poke the sweet potato with a fork. Place in the microwave. Cook for 6 to 8 minutes on high, or until soft and cooked through.

2. In a small bowl, blend together the yogurt, chili powder, paprika, and cumin.

3. In a small pot set over medium heat, heat the olive oil. Add the bell pepper, onion, salt, and pepper. Cook for about 5 minutes, or until the onions have caramelized slightly.

4. Add the edamame. Stir to combine. Cook for 5 minutes more, or until heated through.

5. Slice the potato in half lengthwise.

6. Top each half with half of the edamame mixture, about 2 tablespoons of Cheddar cheese, a dollop of the yogurt mixture, and 2 tablespoons of salsa.

7. Finish with half of the avocado slices and garnish with cilantro.

8. Enjoy!

PER SERVING Calories: 259; Total Fat: 11g; Protein: 15g; Carbohydrates: 33g; Sugars: 7g; Fiber: 9g; Sodium: 417mg

TOSS IT TOGETHER TIP: *Keep a frozen bag of edamame on hand for adding creaminess to smoothies, topping salads, tossing into omelets, using in stir-fries, or making burritos. For a homemade edamame hummus, purée edamame in a food processor with garlic, lemon juice, tahini, and a dash of extra-virgin olive oil.*

Tuna Salad Wraps

QUICK & EASY
PREP TIME: 10 MINUTES

Try something different for lunch. This high-protein, heart-healthy tuna salad comes together in minutes. Deli tuna salad is often mistaken as a healthy choice when it is usually a high-calorie, saturated fat, and sodium-filled bomb. That's because most restaurants are generous with the high-calorie mayonnaise. Here you get all the creamy satisfaction of traditional tuna salad, but it's from high-fiber, heart-healthy avocado and high-protein, calcium-rich Greek yogurt. Calories are kept in check by tucking the salad into lettuce leaves—that's a wrap!

1 (5-ounce) can tuna in water, rinsed and thoroughly drained

1½ teaspoons freshly squeezed lemon juice

½ medium very ripe avocado

2 tablespoons plain nonfat Greek yogurt

¼ cup matchstick carrots

2 radishes, sliced

¼ cup halved green olives

2 tablespoons diced green chiles

1 scallion, diced

Salt, to season

Freshly ground black pepper, to season

2 large green lettuce leaves

1. To a small bowl, add the tuna. Gently flake with a fork. Drizzle with the lemon juice.

2. In a medium bowl, mash the avocado until creamy. Mix in the yogurt.

3. Add the tuna, carrots, radishes, olives, green chiles, and scallion to the avocado mixture. Season with salt and pepper. Stir to combine.

4. Top each lettuce leaf with half of the tuna salad.

5. Wrap and enjoy!

PER SERVING Calories: 178; Total Fat: 7g; Protein: 25g; Carbohydrates: 10g; Sugars: 3g; Fiber: 6g; Sodium: 102mg

TOSS IT TOGETHER TIP: *Leftover green chiles can be used in just about any dish, depending on your personal preferences. Try adding them to omelets, burritos, cooked quinoa, soups, stews, chili, stuffed potatoes, or mixed with your favorite vegetables. Make a Mexican pizza by topping 1 portobello mushroom with Cheddar cheese, chiles, salsa, and avocado slices.*

Nut-Crusted Chicken Fingers

DAIRY-FREE

PREP TIME: 15 MINUTES · COOK TIME: 25 MINUTES

This recipe gives chicken fingers a heart-healthy makeover. The wheat flour and bread crumbs are replaced with almond meal and chopped almonds. Traditional store-bought bread crumbs are made from refined white bread, with high-sodium seasonings, and an array of other ingredients including preservatives. Coating chicken with almond meal not only eliminates questionable ingredients, but adds a delicious, slightly buttery flavor as well as protein, fiber, calcium, potassium, and antioxidants. Additional chopped almonds give the tenders a nice crunch to mimic the crispness you would get by deep frying.

Extra-virgin olive oil cooking spray

½ cup almond meal

¼ cup chopped almonds

1½ teaspoons paprika

½ teaspoon garlic powder

½ teaspoon onion powder

1 teaspoon ground cumin

½ teaspoon dry mustard

½ teaspoon salt

½ teaspoon freshly ground black pepper

8 ounces boneless skinless chicken breasts, sliced into long strips, 1 to 2 inches wide

1 large egg, lightly beaten

1. Preheat the oven to 375°F.

2. Spray a baking sheet with cooking spray. Set aside.

3. In a medium bowl, mix together the almond meal, almonds, paprika, garlic powder, onion powder, cumin, dry mustard, salt, and pepper.

4. Working with one piece of chicken at a time, dredge it in the egg and then coat it with the almond mixture. Place it on the prepared baking sheet. Repeat coating the remaining chicken strips by dredging in the egg first then the almond mixture.

5. Place the sheet in the preheated oven. Bake for 20 to 25 minutes, or until golden.

6. Serve immediately and enjoy!

PER SERVING Calories: 405; Total Fat: 25g; Protein: 38g; Carbohydrates: 9g; Sugars: 1g; Fiber: 4g; Sodium: 90mg

INGREDIENT TIP: *Almond meal is sometimes confused with almond flour. While both products are made from almonds, there is a difference in their consistency and process. Almond meal is coarsely ground unblanched almonds with the outer skin left on. Almond flour is finely ground blanched almonds that have had the skin removed prior to grinding. Store almond meal in the refrigerator to keep it fresh.*

Lazy Turkey Potpie

QUICK & EASY
PREP TIME: 5 MINUTES • COOK TIME: 20 MINUTES

Turkey potpie is classic comfort food and a great one-dish meal. People of all ages love it. And just because it is rich and creamy, and crusty, doesn't mean it's off-limits on a healthy diet. This creative lighter version uses sprouted whole-grain bread for the crust, nonfat dairy products to cut out cholesterol and saturated fats, and low-carbohydrate coconut flour for thickening. Loaded with traditional vegetables, including peas and carrots, this dish is quick and easy to make, and oh-so-satisfying to eat.

2 tablespoons extra-virgin olive oil, divided

½ pound extra-lean ground turkey breast

Salt, to season

Freshly ground black pepper, to season

1 small onion, diced

1 small carrot, diced

½ cup frozen peas

1 teaspoon dried thyme

1 teaspoon dried sage

2 tablespoons coconut flour

2 tablespoons plain nonfat Greek yogurt

1 cup nonfat milk

2 slices sprouted whole-grain bread

1. In a small skillet set over medium heat, heat 1 tablespoon of olive oil.

2. Crumble the turkey in the skillet. Season with salt and pepper. Cook for 5 to 7 minutes, or until no pink color remains. Transfer to a bowl. Set aside.

3. Add the remaining 1 tablespoon of olive oil to the pan. Reduce the heat to low.

4. Add the onion and carrot. Sauté for 5 minutes, or until the vegetables have softened but are not browned.

5. Add the peas. Increase the heat to medium.

6. Sprinkle in the thyme and sage. Stir to combine.

7. Sprinkle the coconut flour over the vegetables. Stir to combine. Cook for 1 minute.

8. Add the yogurt and milk. Season with salt and pepper. Stir to combine. Bring to a simmer. Cook for about 2 minutes, or until thickened.

9. Toast the bread. Slice each piece diagonally. Divide between 2 plates.

10. Top each piece with half of the chicken mixture.

11. Serve immediately and enjoy!

PER SERVING Calories: 461; Total Fat: 17g; Protein: 41g; Carbohydrates: 38g; Sugars: 12g; Fiber: 11g; Sodium: 279mg

INGREDIENT TIP: *Sprouted bread is a great food to include in a healthy carb-controlled diet and makes a great alternative to white flour or whole-grain-flour bread. Sprouting the grains breaks down the proteins and carbohydrates, which makes it easier to digest and lowers the glycemic index. A typical slice of sprouted grain bread has just 80 calories, 11 grams of carbohydrates, 3 grams of fiber, and 4 grams of protein. Keep the bread in the freezer and only take out what you need.*

Cauliflower-Crust Grilled Cheese

PREP TIME: 40 MINUTES • COOK TIME: 10 MINUTES

Recipes for grilled cheese sandwiches date back to ancient Roman texts—and they haven't lost their appeal yet! Comfort food at its best, grilled cheese is a staple in most American homes because it is cheap, fast, and delicious. Unfortunately, grilled cheese is also high in saturated fat, cholesterol, sodium, and carbohydrates. Is there really such a thing as a healthy grilled-cheese sandwich? And, if you don't use bread, is it still a sandwich? This recipe answers both questions with a resounding yes. Cauliflower is creatively made into "bread" slices and nonfat cheese adds the filling. Go on, give it a try! Prepare to be surprised at how delicious and satisfying this "sandwich" really is.

For the cauliflower crust

Extra-virgin olive oil,
    for greasing

1 small cauliflower head, cut
    into florets (about 3 cups)

1 large egg, lighten beaten

½ cup shredded nonfat
    Cheddar cheese

½ teaspoon salt

¼ teaspoon freshly ground
    black pepper

½ teaspoon dry mustard

1 tablespoon nutritional yeast

For the sandwiches

Olive oil cooking spray

⅓ cup nonfat shredded
    Cheddar cheese

To make the cauliflower crust

1. Preheat the oven to 450°F.

2. Place a rack in the middle of the oven.

3. Line a baking sheet with parchment paper. Grease with the olive oil. Set aside.

4. In a food processor, process the cauliflower florets until evenly chopped without being pulverized, until it resembles rice. You should have about 3 cups.

5. Transfer to a microwave-safe dish. Microwave on high for about 8 minutes, or until cooked.

6. In a clean kitchen towel, add the cauliflower rice in the center. Twist the towel around the cauliflower to squeeze out as much moisture as possible. You should get about 1 cup of liquid. The cauliflower rice must be very dry to create the dough. Transfer to a large mixing bowl.

7. Mix in the egg, Cheddar cheese, salt, pepper, dry mustard, and nutritional yeast.

8. Spread the mixture onto the prepared baking sheet. Shape into 4 squares. Place the sheet in the preheated oven. Bake for about 16 minutes, or until golden.

9. Remove from the oven. Cool for 10 minutes. Peel the squares from the parchment, being careful not to break.

To make the sandwiches

1. Spray a large skillet with cooking spray. Place it over medium heat.

2. Lightly coat one side of each slice of "bread" with cooking spray.

3. In the skillet, place 2 "bread" slices, sprayed-side down.

4. Sprinkle half of the Cheddar cheese on each.

5. Top each sandwich with 1 of the 2 remaining "bread" slices, sprayed-side up. Reduce the heat to low.

6. Cook for 2 to 4 minutes, or until golden brown. Gently flip. Cook for 2 to 4 minutes more, until golden brown on the other side.

7. Serve immediately and enjoy!

PER SERVING Calories: 157; Total Fat: 2g; Protein: 21g; Carbohydrates: 10g; Sugars: 3g; Fiber: 3g; Sodium: 365mg

Baked Vegetable Nachos

DAIRY-FREE • QUICK & EASY
PREP TIME: 5 MINUTES • COOK TIME: 10 MINUTES

Health-conscious people typically eat nachos only on rare occasions because many of the usual ingredients are high in unhealthy fats. This dish puts a Mediterranean spin on nachos, using whole-wheat pita bread to make high-fiber baked chips topped with Greek-inspired nutritious toppings. Cucumber, red bell pepper, Kalamata olives, and hummus add protein, fiber, heart-healthy monounsaturated fats, and several servings of vegetables to each portion. Quick and easy to put together, this dish makes a delicious snack, lunch, or side dish.

2 (4-inch) 100 percent whole-wheat pita rounds, quartered and separated into 16 triangles

½ cup quartered grape tomatoes

½ cup diced cucumber

¼ cup diced red bell pepper

2 tablespoons sliced Kalamata olives

4 tablespoons purchased hummus, divided

1. Preheat the oven to 375°F.

2. On a baking sheet, spread the pita pieces in a single layer. Place the sheet in the preheated oven. Bake for 8 to 10 minutes, or until toasted.

3. In a medium bowl, combine the grape tomatoes, cucumber, bell pepper, and olives.

4. Divide the toasted pita between 2 plates.

5. Drop some hummus onto the pita. Spoon the vegetable mixture on top.

6. Serve immediately and enjoy!

PER SERVING Calories: 282; Total Fat: 19g; Protein: 7g; Carbohydrates: 30g; Sugars: 3g; Fiber: 5g; Sodium: 208mg

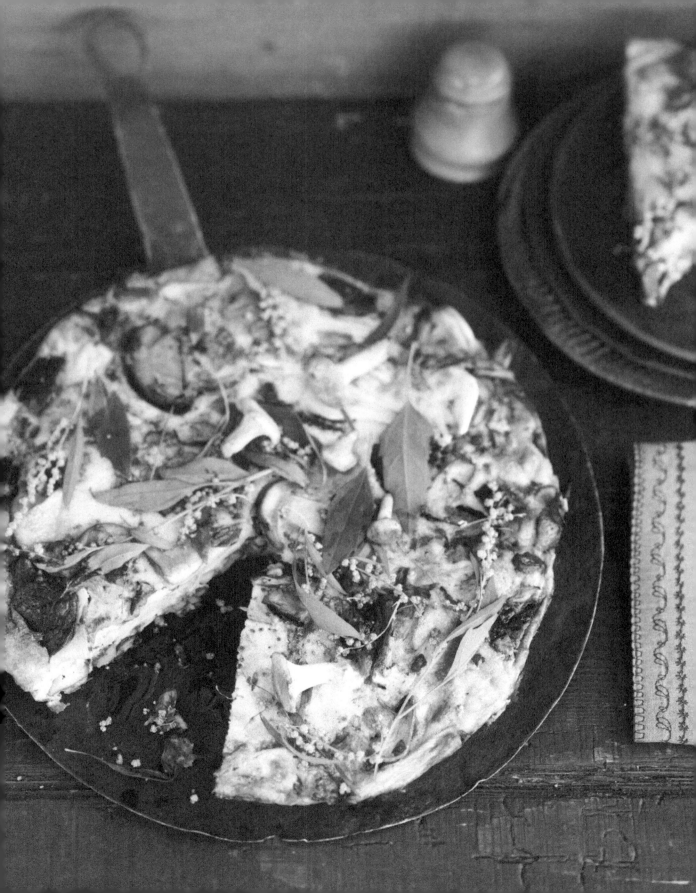

Vegetarian Entrées

Stuffed Acorn Squash

DAIRY-FREE

PREP TIME: 10 MINUTES • COOK TIME: 1 HOUR

Acorn squash is a nutritious fall vegetable, which, unfortunately, is typically cooked with a filling of brown sugar and maple syrup. This recipe uses high-protein quinoa, phytochemical-rich vegetables, and crunchy pistachios to create a convenient dish that even comes in its own serving "bowl."

1 acorn squash, halved and seeded

½ cup water, plus more as needed

¼ cup uncooked quinoa, thoroughly rinsed

1 tablespoon extra-virgin olive oil

¼ cup diced onion

1 garlic clove, chopped

½ cup broccoli florets

½ cup frozen peas

Salt, to season

Freshly ground black pepper, to season

4 tablespoons chopped pistachios, divided

1. Preheat the oven to 425°F.

2. In a large baking dish, place the acorn squash halves cut-side down. Add 1 inch of water to the dish. Place the dish in the preheated oven. Bake for 45 minutes, or until tender.

3. In a small pot set over high heat, bring the water to a boil.

4. Add the quinoa. Reduce the heat to low. Simmer for about 15 minutes, covered, or until tender and all the water is absorbed. Let cool. Fluff with a fork.

5. In a medium saucepan set over medium heat, add the olive oil, onion, and garlic. Sauté for 3 to 4 minutes.

6. Add the broccoli and peas. Cook for about 4 minutes, or until the vegetables are tender.

7. Add the cooked quinoa to the sautéed vegetables. Season with salt and pepper.

8. Spoon half of the mixture into each acorn half.

9. Garnish each half with about 2 tablespoons of pistachios.

10. Serve hot and enjoy!

PER SERVING Calories: 300; Total Fat: 11g; Protein: 9g; Carbohydrates: 45g; Sugars: 4g; Fiber: 8g; Sodium: 67mg

INGREDIENT TIP: *Roast acorn squash seeds by scooping them out, dry on a paper towel, toss with extra-virgin olive oil, and salt, if desired. Preheat the oven to 350°F. Line a baking sheet with parchment paper and spread the seeds in a single layer. Bake for 3 to 5 minutes.*

The Ultimate Veggie Burger

DAIRY-FREE • QUICK & EASY
PREP TIME: 5 MINUTES • COOK TIME: 10 MINUTES

Meat-based burgers are high in unhealthy fats, cholesterol, and sodium. So, swapping that for a vegetarian burger just makes good sense for your health. The problem is that most homemade veggie patties are made from a mix of grains, veggies, and a few beans, so they end up being mostly carbohydrates, not protein. Then, if you put your carb burger on a bun, well, you get the idea. To solve this conundrum, this recipe uses beans, vegetables, and high-protein hemp hearts, which add a nutty flavor and texture for an undeniably delicious vegetarian "burger."

¾ cup shelled edamame

¾ cup frozen mixed vegetables, thawed

3 tablespoons hemp hearts

2 tablespoons quick-cook oatmeal

¼ teaspoon salt

¼ teaspoon onion powder

¼ teaspoon ground cumin

1 scallion, sliced

2 teaspoons chopped fresh cilantro

2 tablespoons coconut flour

2 large egg whites

Extra-virgin olive oil cooking spray

1. In a food processor, combine the edamame, mixed vegetables, hemp hearts, oatmeal, salt, onion powder, cumin, scallion, cilantro, coconut flour, and egg whites. Pulse until blended, but not completely puréed. You want some texture.

2. Spray a nonstick skillet with cooking spray. Place it over medium-high heat.

3. Spoon half of the mixture into the pan. Using the back of a spoon, spread it out to form a patty. Repeat with the remaining half of the mixture.

4. Cook for 3 to 5 minutes, or until golden, and flip. Cook for about 3 minutes more, or until golden. Turn off the heat.

5. Transfer to serving plates and enjoy!

PER SERVING Calories: 303; Total Fat: 10g; Protein: 22g; Carbohydrates: 35g; Sugars: 9g; Fiber: 7g; Sodium: 191mg

TOSS IT TOGETHER TIP: *Hemp seeds, also known as hemp hearts when shelled, are one of the most nutritious seeds you can eat. They are loaded with protein, heart-healthy omega-3 fats, fiber, vitamin E, and minerals like magnesium and zinc. One serving (about 3 tablespoons) contains 11 grams of protein, making them a great food to boost the nutrient power of your diet. Mix them into yogurt and hot cereal, add them to pancakes or scrambled eggs, toss on salads, and sprinkle on steamed vegetables.*

Quinoa–White Bean Loaf

DAIRY-FREE

PREP TIME: 15 MINUTES • COOK TIME: 1 HOUR, 10 MINUTES

One-pot dishes are convenient when cooking for two. In this recipe, a blender makes the prep fast and easy. Beans and high-protein tofu are puréed together and mixed with quinoa and seasonings. Chia seeds and coconut flour bind the ingredients. The result is a creamy, satisfying personal white bean loaf packed with plant-based protein and more than half of your day's fiber requirement. Cook the quinoa in advance for quick assembly.

Extra-virgin olive oil cooking spray

2 teaspoons extra-virgin olive oil

2 garlic cloves, minced

½ cup sliced fresh button mushrooms

6 ounces extra-firm tofu, crumbled

Salt, to season

Freshly ground black pepper, to season

1 (8-ounce) can cannellini beans, drained and rinsed

2 tablespoons coconut flour

1 tablespoon chia seeds

⅓ cup water

½ cup cooked quinoa

¼ cup chopped red onion

¼ cup chopped fresh parsley

1. Preheat the oven to 350°F.

2. Lightly coat 2 mini loaf pans with cooking spray. Set aside.

3. In a large skillet set over medium-high heat, heat the olive oil.

4. Add the garlic, mushrooms, and tofu. Season with salt and pepper.

5. Cook for 6 to 8 minutes, stirring occasionally, until the mushrooms and tofu are golden brown.

6. In a food processor, combine the cannellini beans, coconut flour, chia seeds, and water. Pulse until almost smooth.

7. In a large bowl, mix together the mushroom and tofu mixture, cannellini bean mixture, quinoa, red onion, and parsley. Season with salt and pepper.

8. Evenly divide the mixture between the 2 prepared loaf pans, gently pressing down and mounding the mixture in the middle.

9. Place the pans in the preheated oven. Bake for about 1 hour, or until firm and golden brown. Remove from the oven. Let rest for 10 minutes.

10. Slice and serve.

PER SERVING Calories: 345; Total Fat: 14g; Protein: 21g; Carbohydrates: 43g; Sugars: 2g; Fiber: 14g; Sodium: 142mg

TOSS IT TOGETHER TIP: *This recipe is great for using leftover grains. To cook the quinoa in advance, measure ¼ cup and rinse well under cold water; drain. Put the rinsed quinoa into a saucepan and add ½ cup of cold water. Cover and bring to a boil. As soon as it starts to boil, reduce the heat to a simmer and set the lid ajar to prevent boiling over. Simmer for about 15 minutes, or until the quinoa goes transparent. Fluff with a fork. The proportion of dry quinoa to cooked is a 1:3 ratio, and the quinoa to water ratio is 1:2.*

Lemony Spinach-Tofu Bake

DAIRY-FREE

PREP TIME: 10 MINUTES • COOK TIME: 30 MINUTES

Lemon and marjoram give this dish a wonderfully light, fresh taste, and it couldn't be easier to make. These mini loaves are mixed together in one step and baked. Each ingredient contains an array of health-promoting phytonutrients, making this meal an excellent source of vitamins A and C, and one that is high in protein and low in carbohydrates. For a texture contrast, sliced almonds layer the bottom of the pans and appear as a crunchy topping.

Extra-virgin olive oil cooking spray

1½ cups frozen spinach, thawed and drained

1 cup (about 8 ounces) crumbled firm tofu

½ cup chopped red bell pepper

¼ cup chopped onion

2 tablespoons freshly squeezed lemon juice

1 garlic clove, minced

1 teaspoon dried marjoram

½ teaspoon red pepper flakes

½ cup sliced almonds, divided

1. Preheat the oven to 375°F.

2. Spray 2 mini loaf pans with cooking spray. Set aside.

3. In a medium bowl, mix together the spinach, tofu, bell pepper, onion, lemon juice, garlic, marjoram, and red pepper flakes.

4. Over the bottom of each prepared pan, sprinkle about 2 tablespoons of almonds in a thin layer.

5. Add half of the spinach-tofu mixture to each pan.

6. Top each with about 2 tablespoons of the remaining almonds.

7. Place the pans in the preheated oven. Bake for 30 minutes, or until set.

8. Remove the loaves from the pans and serve immediately.

PER SERVING Calories: 204; Total Fat: 11g; Protein: 15g; Carbohydrates: 13g; Sugars: 4g; Fiber: 4g; Sodium: 128mg

TOSS IT TOGETHER TIP: *Mash leftover tofu and use in place of cottage cheese, add to smoothies for protein, sauté and use as a topping for salads, stir-fry, or scramble for breakfast. You can even freeze tofu for a consistency that makes a great ground beef substitute in pasta sauce and chili.*

Italian Tofu with Mushrooms and Peppers

DAIRY-FREE • QUICK & EASY
PREP TIME: 5 MINUTES • COOK TIME: 10 MINUTES

This aromatic dish can be eaten hot or cold, on its own, or paired with a grain or bean. Tofu is a source of high-quality protein. The portobello mushrooms add a substantial feel from their meaty, chewy texture. This recipe is easy to personalize by adding your favorite vegetables or mixing up the types of mushrooms you use. Leftovers make a great lunch stuffed into a whole-grain pita or topping off a salad with a sprinkle of Parmesan cheese.

1 teaspoon extra-virgin olive oil

¼ cup chopped bell pepper, any color

¼ cup chopped onions

1 garlic clove, minced

8 ounces firm tofu, drained and rinsed

½ cup sliced fresh button mushrooms

1 portobello mushroom cap, chopped

1 tablespoon balsamic vinegar

1 teaspoon dried basil

Salt, to season

Freshly ground black pepper, to season

1. In a medium skillet set over medium heat, heat the olive oil.

2. Add the bell pepper, onions, and garlic. Sauté for 5 minutes, or until soft.

3. Add the tofu, button mushrooms, and portobello mushrooms, tossing and stirring. Reduce the heat to low.

4. Stir in the balsamic vinegar and basil. Season with salt and pepper. Simmer for 2 minutes.

5. Enjoy!

PER SERVING Calories: 129; Total Fat: 6g; Protein: 10g; Carbohydrates: 8g; Sugars: 4g; Fiber: 2g; Sodium: 206mg

TOSS IT TOGETHER TIP: *To minimize waste, purchase frozen chopped bell peppers and diced onions and take out only what you need. If you use fresh vegetables and have leftover bell pepper, toss on salads, add to soups, use to top cooked vegetables, fold into omelets, or garnish a portobello pizza. The same goes for any extra onions, garlic, or mushrooms.*

Asparagus, Sun-Dried Tomato, and Green Pea Sauté

DAIRY-FREE • QUICK & EASY
PREP TIME: 10 MINUTES • COOK TIME: 10 MINUTES

Sautéing is a form of dry-heat cooking that uses a very hot pan and a small amount of fat to cook food very quickly. Sautéing browns the food's surface as it cooks and develops complex flavors and aromas. This simple sauté uses sun-dried tomatoes and tarragon to lend a delicious flavor to this nutritious vegetable mix for a meal that will appeal to multiple senses. For a quick supper or light lunch, serve with a green salad topped with crumbled tofu.

6 packaged sun-dried tomatoes (not packed in oil)

½ cup boiling water

1 tablespoon extra-virgin olive oil

2 garlic cloves, minced

¾ pound fresh asparagus, trimmed and cut into 2-inch pieces

¼ cup chopped red bell pepper

½ cup sliced fresh button mushrooms

¼ cup reduced-sodium vegetable broth

2 tablespoons sliced almonds

1 large tomato, diced (about 1 cup)

1½ teaspoons dried tarragon

½ cup frozen peas

Freshly ground black pepper, to season

1. In a small heatproof bowl, place the sun-dried tomatoes. Cover with the boiling water. Set aside.

2. In a large skillet or wok set over high heat, heat the olive oil.

3. Add the garlic. Swirl in the oil for a few seconds.

4. Toss in the asparagus, red bell pepper, and mushrooms. Stir-fry for 30 seconds.

5. Add the vegetable broth and almonds. Cover and steam for about 2 minutes. Uncover the skillet.

6. Add the tomato and tarragon. Cook for 2 to 3 minutes to reduce the liquid.

7. Drain and chop the sun-dried tomatoes. Add them and the peas to the skillet. Stir-fry for 3 to 4 minutes, or until the vegetables are crisp-tender and the liquid is reduced to a sauce.

8. Season with pepper and serve immediately.

PER SERVING Calories: 221; Total Fat: 11g; Protein: 8g; Carbohydrates: 21g; Sugars: 11g; Fiber: 8g; Sodium: 387mg

TOSS IT TOGETHER TIP: *Use sun-dried tomatoes to flavor omelets, toss with chopped eggplant and herbs served with cheese, toss with sliced fennel, cucumber, and dill for a crunchy side dish, or add to cooked grains and beans.*

Broccoli-Tofu Stir-Fry

DAIRY-FREE • QUICK & EASY
PREP TIME: 5 MINUTES • COOK TIME: 15 MINUTES

A classic vegetarian dish, broccoli and snap peas are quickly stir-fried with tofu for a faster, much healthier dish than most restaurant meals. Chinese five-spice powder brings warm, spicy-sweet flavors to the vegetables and the peanuts add a crunchy finish. If you don't have Chinese five-spice powder, you can make your own. Combine cinnamon, cloves, ginger, ground fennel, and star anise. If you are short on time, use jarred chopped ginger and frozen vegetables. Have all ingredients on hand and prepped before starting.

2 tablespoons extra-virgin olive oil, divided

1 garlic clove, minced

1 tablespoon chopped fresh ginger

8 ounces extra-firm tofu, drained, and cut into 1-inch pieces

2 cups broccoli florets

1 red bell pepper, sliced into strips

1 cup sugar snap peas

1 cup sliced fresh button mushrooms

¼ cup reduced-sodium vegetable broth

1 teaspoon Chinese five-spice powder

1 teaspoon low-sodium soy sauce

2 tablespoons chopped peanuts, divided

2 scallions, chopped, divided

1. In a wok or large skillet set over medium-high heat, heat 1 tablespoon of olive oil.

2. Add the garlic and ginger. Stir-fry for just 30 seconds.

3. Add the tofu. Continue to stir-fry for 3 to 4 minutes, or until the tofu is lightly browned. Transfer the tofu to a bowl. Set aside.

4. To the wok, add the remaining 1 tablespoon of olive oil and heat for a few seconds.

5. Toss in the broccoli, bell pepper, snap peas, and mushrooms. Stir-fry for 1 minute.

6. Pour in the vegetable broth. Stir-fry for 3 minutes more.

7. Add the browned tofu, five-spice powder, and soy sauce. Bring to a simmer. Cook for 4 minutes. Remove from the heat.

8. Evenly portion onto 2 serving plates.

9. Garnish each with 1 tablespoon of peanuts and half of the scallions.

10. Enjoy!

PER SERVING Calories: 350; Total Fat: 25g; Protein: 19g; Carbohydrates: 20g; Sugars: 6g; Fiber: 5g; Sodium: 149mg

Gingered Tofu and Greens

DAIRY-FREE

PREP TIME: 15 MINUTES • COOK TIME: 20 MINUTES

A staple in Asian cooking, bok choy is known for its mild flavor. It is good for stir-fries, braising, and in soups. You can even eat it raw. This vegetable is packed with vitamins A and C, and is very low in calories. Not to be confused with napa cabbage, also a type of Chinese cabbage, bok choy has white stalks that resemble celery, while the dark green, crinkly leaves look similar to romaine lettuce. Stir-fried greens and vegetables are used here as a base for broiled tofu, which is marinated to add flavor. Garnished with hemp hearts, this combination results in a high-protein highly satisfying meal.

For the marinade

2 tablespoons low-sodium
   soy sauce

¼ cup rice vinegar

⅓ cup water

1 tablespoon grated
   fresh ginger

1 tablespoon coconut flour

1 teaspoon granulated stevia

1 garlic clove, minced

To make the marinade

1. In a small bowl, whisk together the soy sauce, rice vinegar, water, ginger, coconut flour, stevia, and garlic until well combined.

2. Place a small saucepan set over high heat. Add the marinade. Bring to a boil. Cook for 1 minute. Remove from the heat.

For the tofu and greens

8 ounces extra-firm
   tofu, drained, cut into
   1-inch cubes

3 teaspoons extra-virgin olive
   oil, divided

1 tablespoon grated
   fresh ginger

2 cups coarsely shredded
   bok choy

2 cups coarsely shredded kale,
   thoroughly washed

½ cup fresh, or frozen,
   chopped green beans

1 tablespoon freshly squeezed
   lime juice

1 tablespoon chopped
   fresh cilantro

2 tablespoons hemp hearts

To make the tofu and greens

1. In a medium ovenproof pan, place the tofu in a single layer. Pour the marinade over. Drizzle with 1½ teaspoons of olive oil. Let sit for 5 minutes.

2. Preheat the broiler to high.

3. Place the pan under the broiler. Broil the tofu for 7 to 8 minutes, or until lightly browned. Using a spatula, turn the tofu over. Continue to broil for 7 to 8 minutes more, or until browned on this side.

4. In a large wok or skillet set over high heat, heat the remaining 1½ teaspoons of olive oil.

5. Stir in the ginger.

6. Add the bok choy, kale, and green beans. Cook for 2 to 3 minutes, stirring constantly, until the greens wilt.

7. Add the lime juice and cilantro. Remove from the heat.

8. Add the browned tofu with any remaining marinade in the pan to the bok choy, kale, and green beans. Toss gently to combine.

9. Top with the hemp hearts and serve immediately.

PER SERVING Calories: 327; Total Fat: 22g; Protein: 21g; Carbohydrates: 19g; Sugars: 3g; Fiber: 8g; Sodium: 613mg

Stuffed Peppers

PREP TIME: 20 MINUTES • COOK TIME: 50 MINUTES

This vegetarian version of stuffed peppers has an Italian flare from the marinara sauce, mozzarella cheese, and basil. Quinoa and tofu add plant-based protein in place of higher-fat ground beef, and walnuts add a rich taste and crunch, as well as heart-healthy omega-3 fats. Portion controlled with no-fuss serving, this healthy dish contains all food groups for a complete meal for two.

½ cup water

¼ cup uncooked quinoa, thoroughly rinsed

1 tablespoon extra-virgin olive oil

1 garlic clove, minced

6 ounces extra-firm tofu, drained and sliced

½ cup marinara sauce, divided

¼ cup finely chopped walnuts

1 teaspoon dried basil

Salt, to season

Freshly ground black pepper, to season

1 red bell pepper, halved and seeded

1 orange bell pepper, halved and seeded

½ cup nonfat shredded mozzarella cheese, divided

4 tomato slices, divided

1. Preheat the oven to 350°F.

2. In a small pot set over high heat, bring the water to a boil.

3. Add the quinoa. Reduce the heat to low. Cover and simmer for about 15 minutes, or until tender and all the water is absorbed. Let cool. Fluff with a fork. Set aside.

4. In a skillet set over medium heat, stir together the olive oil, garlic, and tofu. Cook for about 5 minutes, or until the tofu is evenly brown.

5. Mix in ¼ cup of marinara, the walnuts, and basil. Season with salt and pepper. Cook for 5 minutes more, stirring.

6. Using a wooden spoon or spatula, press one-quarter of the cooked quinoa into each pepper half.

7. Top each with about 1 tablespoon of the remaining ¼ cup of marinara.

8. Sprinkle each with about 1 tablespoon of mozzarella cheese.

9. Place 1 tomato slice on each filled pepper.

10. Finish with about 1 tablespoon of the remaining ¼ cup of mozzarella cheese.

11. Transfer the stuffed peppers to a baking dish. Place the dish in the preheated oven. Bake for 25 minutes, or until the cheese melts.

12. Serve 1 stuffed red bell pepper half and 1 stuffed orange bell pepper half to each person and enjoy!

PER SERVING Calories: 430; Total Fat: 25g; Protein: 26g; Carbohydrates: 30g; Sugars: 8g; Fiber: 7g; Sodium: 423mg

TOSS IT TOGETHER TIP: *Use extra marinara sauce to make chili, creamy tomato soup, or minestrone. Top portobello mushroom caps to make personal pizzas, make Spanish-style rice and beans, dress-up scrambled eggs, or create a tangy vinaigrette to use as a flavorful marinade for grilled meats.*

Edamame Falafel with Roasted Vegetables

DAIRY-FREE
PREP TIME: 10 MINUTES • COOK TIME: 55 MINUTES

Falafel is a traditional Mediterranean dish consisting of deep-fried patties made from chickpeas, fava beans, or both. They are seasoned with cumin and, commonly, served in a pita pocket. This recipe takes a creative spin and uses edamame (green soybeans) for a lighter and creamier falafel than a traditional recipe. Edamame are high in protein and fiber and a good source of iron, vitamin A, and calcium, as well as heart-healthy monounsaturated fats. Paired with a side of roasted vegetables, your taste buds will rejoice at how amazing this meal tastes.

For the roasted vegetables

1 cup broccoli florets

1 medium zucchini, sliced

½ cup cherry
    tomatoes, halved

1½ teaspoons extra-virgin
    olive oil

Salt, to season

Freshly ground black pepper,
    to season

Extra-virgin olive oil
    cooking spray

To make the roasted vegetables

1. Preheat the oven to 425°F.

2. In a large bowl, toss together the broccoli, zucchini, tomatoes, and olive oil to coat. Season with salt and pepper.

3. Spray a baking sheet with cooking spray.

4. Spread the vegetables evenly atop the sheet. Place the sheet in the preheated oven. Roast for 35 to 40 minutes, stirring every 15 minutes, or until the vegetables are soft and cooked through.

5. Remove from the oven. Set aside.

For the falafel

1 cup frozen shelled edamame, thawed

1 small onion, chopped

1 garlic clove, chopped

1 tablespoon freshly squeezed lemon juice

2 tablespoons hemp hearts

1 teaspoon ground cumin

2 tablespoons oat flour

¼ teaspoon salt

Pinch freshly ground black pepper

2 tablespoons extra-virgin olive oil, divided

Prepared hummus, for serving (optional)

To make the falafel

1. In a food processor, pulse the edamame until coarsely ground.

2. Add the onion, garlic, lemon juice, and hemp hearts. Process until finely ground. Transfer the mixture to a medium bowl.

3. By hand, mix in the cumin, oat flour, salt, and pepper.

4. Roll the dough into 1-inch balls. Flatten slightly. You should have about 12 silver dollar–size patties.

5. In a large skillet set over medium heat, heat 1 tablespoon of olive oil.

6. Add 4 falafel patties to the pan at a time (or as many as will fit without crowding), and cook for about 3 minutes on each side, or until lightly browned. Remove from the pan. Repeat with the remaining 1 tablespoon of olive oil and falafel patties.

7. Serve immediately with the roasted vegetables and hummus (if using) and enjoy!

PER SERVING Calories: 356; Total Fat: 22g; Protein: 15g; Carbohydrates: 24g; Sugars: 6g; Fiber: 8g; Sodium: 296mg

TOSS IT TOGETHER TIP: *For even fewer calories, bake the falafel on a sprayed baking sheet. Cook at 375°F for 10 to 15 minutes per side, watching so they don't stick or burn. If you have any leftover falafel, you have a tasty snack, or fold into tortillas or pita for a quick bite, or used as a high-protein topping on a green salad.*

Seitan Curry

DAIRY-FREE
PREP TIME: 10 MINUTES • COOK TIME: 15 MINUTES

Seitan (pronounced *say-tahn*) is a low-fat wheat protein with a chewy texture, making it a great meat substitute. It works so well that many vegetarians avoid it because the texture is too "meaty." Seitan is very versatile. Simmering allows it to soak up the flavor of the herbs and spices used for cooking, so it works well in dishes that utilize sauces, like curries. This dish may reveal a whole new horizon for you in the world of vegetarian cooking.

1 tablespoon extra-virgin olive oil

½ cup chopped onion

2 garlic cloves, chopped

1 cup cauliflower florets

½ cup diced carrots

6 ounces seitan (wheat gluten), finely chopped

2 teaspoons garam masala

1 cup diced tomatoes

⅓ cup unsweetened light canned coconut milk

¼ cup water

Salt, to season

Freshly ground black pepper, to season

2 tablespoons chopped cashews, for garnish

1. In a large wok or skillet set over high heat, heat the olive oil.

2. Add the onion and garlic. Sauté for 3 minutes.

3. Add the cauliflower, carrots, seitan, and garam masala. Mix well. Reduce the heat to medium-high.

4. Stir in the tomatoes, coconut milk, and water. Cover and bring to a simmer. Cook for about 10 minutes, covered, or until the cauliflower and carrots are tender.

5. Season with salt and pepper. Garnish with the cashews.

6. Serve and enjoy!

PER SERVING Calories: 321; Total Fat: 14g; Protein: 24g; Carbohydrates: 23g; Sugars: 7g; Fiber: 3g; Sodium: 514mg

INGREDIENT TIP: *Use canned coconut milk, not the coconut milk beverage in cartons sold in the refrigerated section. Canned coconut milk is made from pressing fresh, ripe coconut milk. You can find unsweetened light coconut milk in the international food section of most grocery stores. Use leftovers in smoothies and cooked hot cereals for extra creaminess.*

Chickpea-Spinach Curry

DAIRY-FREE • QUICK & EASY

PREP TIME: 5 MINUTES • COOK TIME: 10 MINUTES

This recipe is perfect for those days when you are short on time and still want a healthy meal on the table fast. Frozen vegetables and canned beans cut prep time to a bare minimum. Chickpeas are high in fiber, protein, and slow-burning carbohydrates that fuel you up and keep your blood sugar steady. Simply toss the ingredients together, season, simmer, and dinner is served. Serve over high-protein quinoa or with a green salad topped with hemp hearts.

1 cup frozen chopped spinach, thawed

1 cup canned chickpeas, drained and rinsed

½ cup frozen green beans

½ cup frozen broccoli florets

½ cup no-salt-added canned chopped tomatoes, undrained

1 tablespoon curry powder

1 tablespoon granulated garlic

Salt, to season

Freshly ground black pepper, to season

½ cup chopped fresh parsley

1. In a medium saucepan set over high heat, stir together the spinach, chickpeas, green beans, broccoli, tomatoes and their juice, curry powder, and garlic. Season with salt and pepper. Bring to a fast boil. Reduce the heat to low. Cover and simmer for 10 minutes, or until heated through.

2. Top with the parsley, serve, and enjoy!

PER SERVING Calories: 153; Total Fat: 1g; Protein: 10g; Carbohydrates: 28g; Sugars: 3g; Fiber: 11g; Sodium: 190mg

TOSS IT TOGETHER TIP: *Frozen vegetables are just as nutritious as fresh because they are picked and processed at their peak. Keep several bags of different vegetables on hand so you can add a serving or two to all your recipes for additional vitamins, minerals, and fiber.*

Cashew-Kale and Chickpeas

DAIRY-FREE
PREP TIME: 15 MINUTES • COOK TIME: 15 MINUTES

This dish features sautéed kale and beans covered in a rich, decadent-tasting sauce made from cashews. Soaked in water and blended with garlic, the cashews add heart-healthy monounsaturated fats, antioxidants, vitamins, minerals, and their distinctive buttery taste. You'll get plenty of fiber and several servings of vegetables in this high-protein dish—and don't worry about the fat; it's the good kind.

For the cashew sauce

½ cup unsalted cashews soaked in ½ cup hot water for at least 20 minutes

1 cup reduced-sodium vegetable broth

1 garlic clove, minced

For the kale

1 medium red bell pepper, diced

1 medium carrot, julienned

½ cup sliced fresh mushrooms

1 cup canned chickpeas, drained and rinsed

1 bunch kale, thoroughly washed, central stems removed, leaves thinly sliced (about 2½ cups)

2 to 3 tablespoons water

1 teaspoon red pepper flakes

½ teaspoon salt

Freshly ground black pepper, to season

¼ cup minced fresh cilantro

To make the cashew sauce

1. Drain the cashews.

2. In a blender or food processor, blend together the cashews, vegetable broth, and garlic until completely smooth. Set aside.

To make the kale

1. In a large nonstick skillet or Dutch oven set over medium-low heat, stir together the red bell pepper, carrot, and mushrooms. Cook for 5 to 7 minutes, or until softened.

2. Stir in the chickpeas. Increase the heat to high.

3. Add the kale and the water. Stir to combine. Cover and cook for 5 minutes, or until the kale is tender.

4. Stir in the cashew sauce, red pepper flakes, and salt. Season with pepper. Cook for 2 to 3 minutes more, uncovered, or until the sauce thickens.

5. Garnish with the cilantro before serving.

6. Enjoy!

PER SERVING Calories: 348; Total Fat: 15g; Protein: 16g; Carbohydrates: 45g; Sugars: 5g; Fiber: 13g; Sodium: 408mg

RECIPE TIP: *If you don't have fresh greens on hand, use a 10-ounce package of frozen kale, or other hardy green, like collards. You can also use frozen bell peppers. Just measure out the amount you need without worrying about waste.*

Grilled Vegetables on White Bean Mash

DAIRY-FREE
PREP TIME: 15 MINUTES • COOK TIME: 30 MINUTES

If you are looking for something different to serve with vegetables that is lower in carbs than pasta, rice, or potatoes, try mashed beans. With the consistency of mashed potatoes or polenta and the heartiness of legumes, this dish makes an unexpected and yet incredibly satisfying side for grilled vegetables. It's super easy and quick to prepare with canned beans, and you can use any vegetables you have on hand. Enjoy served over fresh baby spinach.

2 medium zucchini, sliced

1 red bell pepper, seeded and quartered

2 portobello mushroom caps, quartered

3 teaspoons extra-virgin olive oil, divided

1 (8-ounce) can cannellini beans, drained and rinsed

1 garlic clove, minced

½ cup low-sodium vegetable broth

4 cups baby spinach, divided

Salt, to season

Freshly ground black pepper, to season

1 tablespoon chopped fresh parsley

2 lemon wedges, divided, for garnish

1. Preheat the grill. Use a stove-top grill pan or broiler if a grill is not available.

2. Lightly brush the zucchini, red bell pepper, and mushrooms with 1½ teaspoons of olive oil. Arrange them in a barbecue grill pan. Place the pan on the preheated grill. Cook the vegetables for 5 to 8 minutes, or until lightly browned. Turn the vegetables. Brush with the remaining 1½ teaspoons of olive oil. Cook for 5 to 8 minutes more, or until tender.

3. To a small pan set over high heat, add the cannellini beans, garlic, and vegetable broth. Bring to a boil. Reduce the heat to low. Simmer for 10 minutes, uncovered. Using a potato masher, roughly mash the beans, adding a little more broth if they seem too dry.

4. Place 2 cups of spinach on each serving plate.

5. Top each with half of the bean mash and half of the grilled vegetables. Season with salt and pepper. Garnish with parsley.

6. Place 1 lemon wedge on each plate and serve.

PER SERVING Calories: 244; Total Fat: 8g; Protein: 13g; Carbohydrates: 35g; Sugars: 9g; Fiber: 6g; Sodium: 241mg

TOSS IT TOGETHER TIP: *Keep cubes of low-sodium vegetable broth in your pantry so you can prepare only what you need for each recipe. If you prefer the boxed or canned broth, use leftovers in soups, to simmer vegetables, to cook beans, or to make a marinade for fish, chicken, or tofu.*

Lentil and Cheese Burritos

PREP TIME: 15 MINUTES • COOK TIME: 30 MINUTES

The mighty lentil creates an energy-packed low-carb burrito that will fill you up without loading you down with carbs. Lentils are a powerhouse of nutrition. Lower in calories and higher in protein than other beans, lentils balance blood-sugar levels and provide steady energy from their high fiber content. Cooked with plenty of vegetables and wrapped in a low-carb whole-wheat tortilla, this dish can be eaten for breakfast, lunch, or dinner.

1 cup water

⅓ cup lentils, thoroughly rinsed

2 teaspoons extra-virgin olive oil

¼ cup diced onion

1 garlic clove, minced

1 cup chopped zucchini

½ teaspoon ground cumin

½ cup salsa

Salt, to season

Freshly ground black pepper, to season

½ cup shredded nonfat Cheddar cheese

2 (7-inch) 100 percent whole-wheat low-carb tortillas, divided

½ cup shredded lettuce, divided

1. In a medium pot set over high heat, bring the water to a boil.

2. Add the lentils. Reduce the heat to low. Cover and simmer for about 20 minutes, or until just tender. Drain, if necessary. Set aside.

3. In a medium skillet set over medium heat, heat the olive oil.

4. Add the onion, garlic, and zucchini. Sauté for about 5 minutes, or until tender.

5. Stir in the cooked lentils, cumin, and salsa. Season with salt and pepper. Simmer for 5 minutes.

6. Stir in the Cheddar cheese. Remove from the heat.

7. Place 1 tortilla on each serving plate. Top with ¼ cup of shredded lettuce and half of the lentil mixture.

8. Roll up and enjoy!

PER SERVING Calories: 237; Total Fat: 7g; Protein: 23g; Carbohydrates: 37g; Sugars: 7g; Fiber: 18g; Sodium: 697mg

RECIPE TIP: *Serve this burrito in lettuce leaves for an even lower-carb meal. Choose large, crisp, fresh romaine lettuce leaves. Wash the leaves thoroughly and pat dry with a paper towel before using to remove excess moisture.*

Cheesy Zucchini Patties

QUICK & EASY

PREP TIME: 10 MINUTES • COOK TIME: 20 MINUTES

These vegetable patties are so easy to make and so delicious to eat! Plus, you can customize this recipe based on whatever vegetables you have on hand. The ground flaxseed and egg bind the ingredients together, and the cheese makes them creamy, gooey, and satisfying. Cook these little patties like you would a pancake, on a griddle or in a sauté pan. For a complete meal on their own, serve on a bed of mixed baby greens.

1 cup grated zucchini

1 cup chopped
    fresh mushrooms

½ cup grated carrot

½ cup nonfat shredded
    mozzarella cheese

¼ cup finely ground flaxseed

1 large egg, beaten

1 garlic clove, minced

Salt, to season

Freshly ground black pepper,
    to season

1 tablespoon extra-virgin
    olive oil

4 cup mixed baby
    greens, divided

1. In a medium bowl, stir together the zucchini, mushrooms, carrot, mozzarella cheese, flaxseed, egg, and garlic. Season with salt and pepper. Stir again to combine.

2. In a large skillet set over medium-high heat, heat the olive oil.

3. Drop 1 tablespoon of the zucchini mixture into the skillet. Continue dropping tablespoon-size portions in the pan until it is full, but not crowded. Cook for 2 to 3 minutes on each side, or until golden. Transfer to a serving plate. Repeat with the remaining mixture.

4. Place 2 cups of greens on each serving plate. Top each with zucchini patties.

5. Enjoy!

PER SERVING Calories: 297; Total Fat: 13g; Protein: 22g; Carbohydrates: 23g; Sugars: 13g; Fiber: 12g; Sodium: 880mg

TOSS IT TOGETHER TIP: *Use any vegetable you like in this recipe. It is perfect for using what's on hand that may be close to spoiling. Try different types of cheese or substitute mashed tofu for a different texture and taste. Use your favorite seasonings, mix in fresh herbs, or add a few chopped nuts for a texture contrast.*

Sautéed Spinach and Lima Beans

DAIRY-FREE
PREP TIME: 5 MINUTES • COOK TIME: 40 MINUTES

Frozen lima beans get a spicy kick from a dash of cayenne. Lima beans are an excellent source of fiber, phytochemicals, antioxidants, vitamins, minerals, and plant sterols. Combined with nutrient-rich spinach, this dish is rich in cholesterol-lowering nutrients, as well as plant-based protein. Nourishing and delicious, this makes a light supper on a busy weeknight.

Extra-virgin olive oil cooking spray

¼ cup chopped onion

½ cup low-sodium vegetable broth

1 cup frozen lima beans, thawed

2 teaspoons extra-virgin olive oil

2 garlic cloves, chopped

4 cups chopped fresh spinach

Pinch cayenne pepper

2 teaspoons balsamic vinegar

Salt, to season

Freshly ground black pepper, to season

1. Heat a large saucepan over medium heat. Spray with cooking spray.

2. Add the onion. Sauté for about 4 minutes, or until soft and translucent.

3. Add the vegetable broth. Bring to a boil.

4. Add the lima beans and just enough water to cover. Bring to a boil. Reduce the heat to low. Cover and simmer for 30 minutes, or until the beans are tender. Set aside.

5. Heat a large skillet over medium-high heat for 30 seconds.

6. Add the olive oil and garlic. Sauté for 1 to 2 minutes, or until golden. Remove the garlic and reserve.

7. To the skillet, add the spinach and cayenne. Cover and cook for about 1 minute, or until the leaves wilt. Drain to remove any excess water.

8. Stir in the balsamic vinegar. Season with salt and pepper.

9. To serve, mound half of the spinach on a plate, top with half of the lima beans, and sprinkle with the reserved garlic.

PER SERVING Calories: 188; Total Fat: 4g; Protein: 9g; Carbohydrates: 27g; Sugars: 4g; Fiber: 7g; Sodium: 348mg

Soybeans with Plums and Peppers

DAIRY-FREE
PREP TIME: 15 MINUTES • COOK TIME: 40 MINUTES

Plums add an exotic taste to this savory dish that also contains black soybeans and peppers. Black soybeans are a great addition to a low-carb pantry and a great substitute for higher-carb beans. Nutritionally, they have more protein per serving than most other beans, and their high fiber content means they are low in net carbohydrates. Rich in phytonutrients, antioxidants, vitamin K, iron, and magnesium, they provide a powerful plant-based punch of protein in this deliciously creative recipe.

2 medium purple plums

1 tablespoon extra-virgin olive oil

1 medium onion, chopped

1 small yellow bell pepper, chopped

1 small red bell pepper, chopped

1 garlic clove, chopped

2 whole cloves

2 teaspoons ground cumin

½ cup minced fresh cilantro leaves

2 teaspoons freshly squeezed lemon juice

½ teaspoon liquid stevia

1 cup cooked black soybeans

1. Fill a deep pot with water and bring to a boil over high heat.

2. Add the plums. Boil for 30 seconds to loosen their skins. With a slotted spoon, remove the plums. Set aside to cool.

3. In a large skillet set over low heat, heat the olive oil.

4. Add the onion, yellow bell pepper, red bell pepper, garlic, whole cloves, cumin, and cilantro. Cook for 5 to 10 minutes, stirring frequently, until the onion softens.

5. Peel the plums. Remove the pits and chop the fruit.

6. Add the plum, lemon juice, and stevia to the onions and peppers.

7. Stir in the black soybeans. Cover and cook for about 30 minutes, or until the peppers are soft, stirring frequently to prevent sticking.

8. Remove the 2 whole cloves. Serve hot or chilled and enjoy!

PER SERVING Calories: 467; Total Fat: 23g; Protein: 31g; Carbohydrates: 44g; Sugars: 17g; Fiber: 23g; Sodium: 7mg

INGREDIENT TIP: *Most health food stores carry canned organic black soybeans by Eden Foods. You can also find them dried. Use leftovers to make low-carb baked beans, refried beans, bean soup, chili, four-bean salad, or process into a paste with garlic and onion for a healthy dip or spread.*

Black-Eyed Pea Sauté with Garlic and Olives

DAIRY-FREE • QUICK & EASY
PREP TIME: 5 MINUTES • COOK TIME: 5 MINUTES

Black-eyed peas, a legume, are well known in Southern cooking, but their nutritional content makes them an excellent addition to any menu. Low in calories and high in fiber, protein, and essential vitamins and minerals, black-eyed peas are considered to have a very low glycemic index. This simple yet tasty sauté pairs the distinctive taste and heart-healthy oils of Kalamata olives with black-eyed peas and thyme. Satisfying on its own, this dish also works well with baked tofu, chicken, or fish.

2 teaspoons extra-virgin olive oil

1 garlic clove, minced

½ red onion, chopped

1 cup cooked black-eyed peas; if canned, drain and rinse

½ teaspoon dried thyme

¼ cup water

¼ teaspoon salt

¼ teaspoon freshly ground black pepper

6 Kalamata olives, pitted and halved

1. In a medium saucepan set over medium heat, stir together the olive oil, garlic, and red onion. Cook for 2 minutes, continuing to stir.

2. Add the black-eyed peas and thyme. Cook for 1 minute.

3. Stir in the water, salt, pepper, and olives. Cook for 2 minutes more, or until heated through.

PER SERVING Calories: 198; Total Fat: 9g; Protein: 7g; Carbohydrates: 22g; Sugars: 4g; Fiber: 6g; Sodium: 237mg

INGREDIENT TIP: *You can find fresh black-eyed peas year-round in the produce section of most grocery stores. They are also sold canned and frozen. Choose the option that works best for you. Presoaking is not essential when cooking fresh black-eyed peas, but they will require about 1 hour to cook.*

Easy Cheesy Vegetable Frittata

QUICK & EASY
PREP TIME: 10 MINUTES • COOK TIME: 15 MINUTES

A frittata is an Italian egg-based dish similar to an omelet, without the trickiness of the flip. Having a good frittata recipe in your repertoire is an incredibly useful thing. When you need a quick and satisfying protein-rich meal, there are few things more satisfying. Frittatas are quick and easy to prepare and customizable to the vegetables you have on hand. Simply add a green salad and you are good to go.

Extra-virgin olive oil
   cooking spray
½ cup sliced onion
½ cup sliced green
   bell pepper
½ cup sliced eggplant
½ cup frozen spinach
½ cup sliced
   fresh mushrooms
1 tablespoon chopped
   fresh basil
Pinch freshly ground
   black pepper
½ cup liquid egg substitute
½ cup nonfat cottage cheese
¼ cup fat-free
   evaporated milk
¼ cup nonfat shredded
   Cheddar cheese

1. Coat an ovenproof 10-inch skillet with cooking spray. Place it over medium-low heat until hot.

2. Add the onion, green bell pepper, eggplant, spinach, and mushrooms. Sauté for 2 to 3 minutes, or until lightly browned.

3. Add the basil. Season with pepper. Stir to combine. Cook for 2 to 3 minutes more, or until the flavors blend. Remove from the heat.

4. Preheat the broiler.

5. In a blender, combine the egg substitute, cottage cheese, Cheddar cheese, and evaporated milk. Process until smooth. Pour the egg mixture over the vegetables in the skillet.

6. Return the skillet to medium-low heat. Cover and cook for about 5 minutes, or until the bottom sets and the top is still slightly wet.

7. Transfer the ovenproof skillet to the broiler. Broil for 2 to 3 minutes, or until the top is set.

8. Serve one-half of the frittata per person and enjoy!

PER SERVING Calories: 168; Total Fat: 0.5g; Protein: 23g; Carbohydrates: 16g; Sugars: 10g; Fiber: 4g; Sodium: 594mg

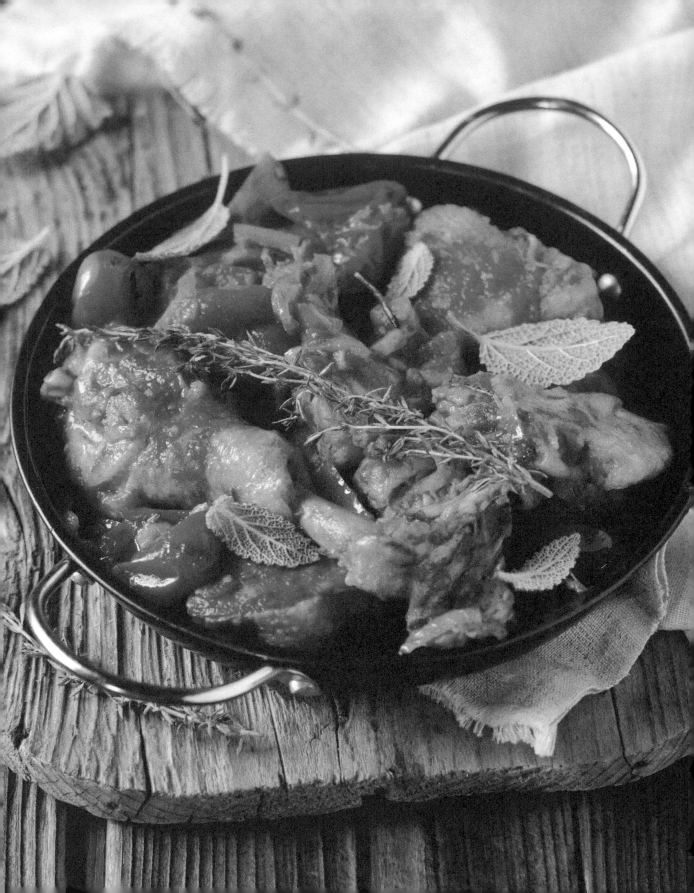

CHAPTER 8

Chicken & Fish Entrées

Kung Pao Chicken and Zucchini Noodles

DAIRY-FREE • QUICK & EASY

PREP TIME: 15 MINUTES • COOK TIME: 15 MINUTES

Finally, you can enjoy the distinctive, rich flavors of Kung Pao Noodles without all of the guilt. This recipe replaces high-carb egg noodles with low-calorie, high-fiber zucchini noodles. Each serving, filled with chicken and several servings of vegetables, has a flavor combination that includes salty, sweet, sour, and spicy. Topped with crushed peanuts, this dish is as nutritious as it is delicious, and hard to pass up. You just may never order takeout again.

For the noodles

2 medium zucchini,
    ends trimmed

For the sauce

1½ tablespoons low-sodium
    soy sauce

1 tablespoon balsamic vinegar

1 teaspoon hoisin sauce

2½ tablespoons water

1½ teaspoons red chili paste

2 teaspoons granulated stevia

2 teaspoons cornstarch

To make the noodles

With a spiralizer or julienne peeler, cut the zucchini lengthwise into spaghetti-like strips. Set aside.

To make the sauce

In a small bowl, whisk together the soy sauce, balsamic vinegar, hoisin sauce, water, red chili paste, stevia, and cornstarch. Set aside.

For the chicken

6 ounces boneless skinless
   chicken breast, cut into
   ½-inch pieces

Salt, to season

Freshly ground black pepper,
   to season

1 teaspoon extra-virgin
   olive oil

1 teaspoon sesame oil

2 garlic cloves, minced

1 tablespoon chopped
   fresh ginger

½ red bell pepper, cut into
   ½-inch pieces

½ (8-ounce) can water
   chestnuts, drained
   and sliced

1 celery stalk, cut into
   ¾-inch dice

2 tablespoons crushed dry-
   roasted peanuts, divided

2 tablespoons
   scallions, divided

To make the chicken

1. Season the chicken with salt and pepper.

2. In a large, deep nonstick pan or wok set over medium-high heat, heat the olive oil.

3. Add the chicken. Cook for 4 to 5 minutes, stirring, or until browned and cooked through. Transfer the chicken to a plate. Set aside.

4. Return the pan to the stove. Reduce the heat to medium.

5. Add the sesame oil, garlic, and ginger. Cook for about 30 seconds, or until fragrant.

6. Add the red bell pepper, water chestnuts, and celery.

7. Stir in the sauce. Bring to a boil. Reduce the heat to low. Simmer for 1 to 2 minutes, until thick and bubbling.

8. Stir in the zucchini noodles. Cook for about 2 minutes, tossing, until just tender and mixed with the sauce.

9. Add the chicken and any accumulated juices. Stir to combine. Cook for about 2 minutes, or until heated through.

10. Divide the mixture between 2 bowls. Top each serving with 1 tablespoon of peanuts and 1 tablespoon of scallions. Enjoy!

PER SERVING Calories: 335; Total Fat: 11g; Protein: 26g; Carbohydrates: 34g; Sugars: 12g; Fiber: 5g; Sodium: 595mg

INGREDIENT TIP: *Water chestnuts belong to the non-starchy, low-calorie vegetable group that can keep you fuller longer, while adding valuable B vitamins and minerals to meals. Water chestnuts have just 60 calories per ½-cup serving, so don't worry about eating more of this nutritious vegetable if watching your weight. Add to salads, soups, wraps, or as a pizza topping.*

Chicken Parmesan

PREP TIME: 30 MINUTES • COOK TIME: 1 HOUR

Classic chicken Parmesan, referred to colloquially as "chicken parm," gets a makeover that uses nutrient-rich almond meal in place of traditional bread crumbs, nonfat mozzarella, and—if you dare—soy Parmesan. The cooking process is the same as when making traditional chicken Parmesan and the result is equally delicious. This is sure to be one of those "I want this tonight" recipe favorites.

Extra-virgin olive oil cooking spray

1 large egg

¼ cup almond meal

2 (6-ounce) boneless skinless chicken breast halves

1 (8-ounce) jar marinara sauce, divided

4 tablespoons nonfat shredded mozzarella cheese, divided

4 tablespoons grated non-dairy soy Parmesan cheese, divided

4 tablespoons chopped fresh basil, divided

Salt, to season

Freshly ground black pepper, to season

1. Preheat the oven to 350°F.

2. Lightly coat a baking sheet with cooking spray.

3. In a shallow bowl, beat the egg.

4. In a separate shallow bowl, place the almond meal.

5. Dip 1 chicken breast half into the egg, then into the almond meal to coat. Place the coated chicken on the prepared baking sheet. Repeat with the remaining 1 chicken breast half.

6. Place the sheet in the preheated oven. Bake for 40 minutes, or until no longer pink and the juices run clear.

7. In a baking dish, pour 4 ounces of marinara sauce.

8. Place the cooked chicken on the sauce. Cover with the remaining 4 ounces of marinara.

9. Sprinkle 2 tablespoons of mozzarella cheese and 2 tablespoons of soy Parmesan cheese on each chicken breast. Top each with 2 tablespoons of basil.

10. Place the dish in the oven. Bake for 20 minutes, or until an instant-read thermometer inserted into the center reads at least 165°F.

11. Remove from oven and divide between 2 plates. Season with salt and pepper and enjoy!

PER SERVING Calories: 393; Total Fat: 15g; Protein: 56g; Carbohydrates: 12g; Sugars: 0g; Fiber: 1g; Sodium: 919mg

Lemon-Herb Chicken

DAIRY-FREE · QUICK & EASY
PREP TIME: 10 MINUTES · COOK TIME: 20 MINUTES

It doesn't get much easier, or more satisfying, than this simple recipe that's on the table in about 30 minutes. Lemon brightens the chicken's flavor and tenderizes it so it's juicy and moist—with just the right amount of tartness. Serve with a side of roasted root vegetables, a green salad, and brown rice.

1 lemon, halved, divided

2 (6-ounce) boneless skinless chicken breast halves

Salt, to season

1 tablespoon extra-virgin olive oil

2 garlic cloves, minced

¼ cup finely chopped sweet onion

Freshly ground black pepper, to season

1 teaspoon dried oregano

2 sprigs fresh parsley

1. Squeeze the juice from 1 lemon half over the chicken. Season with salt. Set aside.

2. In a small skillet set over medium low heat, heat the olive oil.

3. Add the garlic and onion. Sauté the garlic and onion. Add the chicken to the skillet. As it cooks, squeeze the juice from the remaining lemon half over the chicken. Season with salt and pepper. Sprinkle with the oregano. Sauté for 5 to 10 minutes per side, or until the juices run clear.

4. Serve garnished with the parsley.

PER SERVING Calories: 280; Total Fat: 13g; Protein: 38g; Carbohydrates: 2g; Sugars: 0g; Fiber: 0g; Sodium: 63mg

INGREDIENT TIP: *It can be difficult to find small chicken breasts. Remove the strip of meat from the underside of a 5- to 6-ounce breast, which is the "tender"—about 1 ounce of meat, to yield a perfect individual portion. Freeze the tenders and use in a stir-fry.*

Easy Chicken Cacciatore

DAIRY-FREE • QUICK & EASY
PREP TIME: 5 MINUTES • COOK TIME: 20 MINUTES

Chicken cacciatore is an Italian dish of chicken braised in a tomato-based sauce that often includes wild mushrooms. It is frequently referred to as "hunter style," as the word *cacciatore* means "hunter" in Italian. Why "hunter" style? One story says if a hunter came home empty-handed, his wife would kill a chicken for the meal instead. This hunter-style dish makes good use of mushrooms, onions, tomatoes, and herbs. Enjoy over a bed of spaghetti squash "noodles."

Extra-virgin olive oil cooking spray

1 garlic clove, chopped

½ cup chopped red onion

¾ cup chopped green bell pepper

2 (6-ounce) boneless skinless chicken breasts, cubed

1 cup sliced cremini mushrooms

½ cup chopped tomatoes, with juice

1 cup green beans

1 teaspoon dried oregano

1 teaspoon dried rosemary

1. Coat a skillet with cooking spray. Place it over medium heat.

2. Add the garlic. Sauté for about 1 minute, or until browned.

3. Add the red onion, green bell pepper, and chicken. Cook for about 6 minutes, or until the chicken is slightly browned, tossing to cook all sides.

4. Stir in the mushrooms, tomatoes, green beans, oregano, and rosemary. Reduce the heat to medium-low. Simmer for 8 to 10 minutes, stirring constantly.

5. Remove from the heat and serve hot.

6. Enjoy!

PER SERVING Calories: 292; Total Fat: 6g; Protein: 42g; Carbohydrates: 13g; Sugars: 5g; Fiber: 3g; Sodium: 69mg

Chicken Cordon Bleu

QUICK & EASY

PREP TIME: 10 MINUTES • COOK TIME: 15 MINUTES

A delicious French classic, this chicken *cordon bleu* (translated literally as "blue ribbon") is easy to prepare and lighter in calories and fat than traditional recipes. Almond meal replaces bread crumbs to cut down on carbs, while adding vitamin E and heart-healthy fats. Good for you and delicious, you'll award yourself the "blue ribbon" of culinary excellence after making this dish.

2 (6-ounce) boneless skinless chicken breasts, trimmed, tenders removed

⅛ teaspoon salt

¼ teaspoon freshly ground black pepper, divided

3 tablespoons nonfat shredded Swiss cheese

1 tablespoon plain nonfat Greek yogurt

2 tablespoons almond meal

2 teaspoons chopped fresh parsley

1 teaspoon dried thyme

2 **teaspoons extra-virgin olive oil, divided**

2 tablespoons (about ½ ounce) chopped ham

1. Preheat the oven to 400°F.

2. Sprinkle the chicken with the salt and ⅛ teaspoon of pepper.

3. In a small bowl, stir together the Swiss cheese and yogurt.

4. In another small bowl, stir together the remaining ⅛ teaspoon of pepper, the almond meal, parsley, thyme, and 1 teaspoon of olive oil.

5. In a medium ovenproof nonstick skillet set over medium heat, heat the remaining 1 teaspoon of olive oil.

6. Add the chicken. Cook for about 2 minutes per side, or until browned. Move the chicken to the center of the skillet, so the pieces touch.

7. Spread the chicken with the cheese mixture, sprinkle with the ham, and top with the seasoned almond meal.

8. Place the ovenproof skillet in the preheated oven. Bake for 5 to 7 minutes, or until the chicken is no longer pink in the center and an instant-read thermometer registers 165°F.

9. Bon appétit!

PER SERVING Calories: 339; Total Fat: 15g; Protein: 48g; Carbohydrates: 3g; Sugars: 2g; Fiber: 0g; Sodium: 302mg

Roast Chicken with Pine Nuts and Fennel

DAIRY-FREE

PREP TIME: 20 MINUTES · COOK TIME: 30 MINUTES

With Italian spices, toasty pine nuts, and aromatic fennel bulb, you have a hearty and superbly satisfying gourmet meal that's ready in a flash. Skinless chicken drumsticks are rubbed with an herb paste, roasted with fennel and mixed vegetables, and topped with crunchy pine nuts to create a mouthwatering dish. Fennel bulb has a unique array of phytonutrients, is high in vitamin C, cholesterol-lowering fiber, potassium, and B vitamins that support heart health. Enjoy this recipe with a simple salad.

For the herb paste

2 tablespoons fresh rosemary leaves

1 tablespoon freshly grated lemon zest

2 garlic cloves, quartered

½ teaspoon freshly ground black pepper

¼ teaspoon salt

1 teaspoon extra-virgin olive oil

For the chicken

4 (6-ounce) skinless chicken drumsticks

2 teaspoons extra-virgin olive oil

To make the herb paste

1. On a cutting board, combine the rosemary, lemon zest, garlic, pepper, and salt. Mince into a fine paste. Transfer to a small bowl.

2. Stir in the olive oil.

To make the chicken

1. Rub the herb paste over the drumsticks. Set aside.

2. In a large nonstick skillet set over medium-high heat, heat the olive oil.

3. Add the coated drumsticks. Cook for 4 to 5 minutes, turning occasionally, until browned on all sides. Remove from the heat and keep warm.

For the vegetables

1 large fennel bulb, cored and chopped (about 3 cups)

1 cup sliced fresh mushrooms

½ cup sliced carrots

¼ cup chopped sweet onion

2 teaspoons extra-virgin olive oil

2 tablespoons pine nuts

2 teaspoons white wine vinegar

To make the vegetables

1. Preheat the oven to 450°F.

2. In a 9-by-13-inch baking dish, toss together the fennel, mushrooms, carrots, onion, and olive oil. Place the dish in the preheated oven. Bake for 10 minutes.

3. Stir in the pine nuts.

4. Top with the browned drumsticks. Return the dish to the oven. Bake for 15 to 20 minutes more, or until the fennel is golden and an instant-read thermometer inserted into the thickest part of a drumstick without touching the bone registers 165°F.

5. Remove the chicken from the pan.

6. Stir the white wine vinegar into the pan. Toss the vegetables to coat, scraping up any browned bits.

7. Serve the chicken with the vegetables and enjoy!

PER SERVING Calories: 505; Total Fat: 23g; Protein: 31g; Carbohydrates: 22g; Sugars: 4g; Fiber: 6g; Sodium: 702mg

Crispy Baked Drumsticks with Mustard Sauce

PREP TIME: 15 MINUTES • COOK TIME: 30 MINUTES

Fried chicken is loaded with unhealthy fats, is high in calories, and doesn't really fit in a healthy eating plan—but it tastes good. So, this recipe lets you enjoy the taste without worrying about harming your health. The traditional breading is replaced with almond meal and the dish is baked instead of fried. Topping it all off is a low-sugar but tasty mustard sauce. Enjoy with a side of steamed broccoli and a green salad.

For the chicken

Extra-virgin olive oil cooking spray

⅓ cup almond meal

¼ teaspoon paprika

¼ teaspoon onion powder

¼ teaspoon salt

2 teaspoons extra-virgin olive oil

1 large egg

4 (4-ounce) skinless chicken drumsticks, trimmed

For the mustard sauce

2 tablespoons plain nonfat Greek yogurt

1 tablespoon Dijon mustard

¼ teaspoon liquid stevia

Freshly ground black pepper, to season

To make the chicken

1. Preheat the oven to 475°F.

2. Coat a wire rack with cooking spray. Place the rack on a large rimmed baking sheet.

3. In a shallow dish, stir together the almond meal, paprika, onion powder, and salt. Drizzle with the olive oil. Mash together with a fork until the oil is thoroughly incorporated.

4. In another shallow dish, lightly beat the egg with a fork.

5. Working with 1 drumstick at a time, dip each into the egg, then press into the almond meal mixture, coating evenly on both sides. Place the chicken on the prepared rack. Repeat until all pieces are coated.

6. Place the sheet in the preheated oven. Bake for 25 to 30 minutes, or until golden and an instant-read thermometer inserted into the thickest part of a drumstick without touching the bone registers 165°F.

To make the mustard sauce

1. In a small bowl, stir together the yogurt, mustard, and stevia. Season with pepper.

2. Serve the sauce with the drumsticks.

PER SERVING Calories: 363; Total Fat: 15g; Protein: 30g; Carbohydrates: 5g; Sugars: 0g; Fiber: 0g; Sodium: 46mg

Blackened Pollock

DAIRY-FREE • QUICK & EASY
PREP TIME: 15 MINUTES • COOK TIME: 10 MINUTES

You don't need to fire up the grill to make this nutritious and tasty Cajun blackened-pollock dish. Blackening is a cooking technique for which meat is covered in spices and cooked over very high heat. The spices used turn black easily and impart great flavor, resulting in a blackened exterior and an interior cooked to your taste. Serve with a side of black-eyed peas for a truly Cajun-inspired meal.

8 ounces Pollock (or other white fish) fillet, skinned and halved

3 teaspoons extra-virgin olive oil, divided

1 teaspoon blackening seasoning, or Cajun seasoning, divided

¼ cup thinly sliced onion

4 cups baby spinach, divided

½ small grapefruit, peeled and segmented

2 tablespoons shaved fennel

2 tablespoons pepitas

½ small avocado, peeled, pitted, and sliced, divided

1. Brush both sides of each pollock half with 1½ teaspoons of olive oil.

2. Rub each half all over with ½ teaspoon of blackening seasoning.

3. In a large heavy skillet set over high heat, cook the pollock and onions for 2 to 3 minutes, until blackened. Turn the fillets. Cook for 2 to 3 minutes more, or until blackened and the fish flakes easily with a fork.

4. Put 2 cups of arugula on each serving plate. Top each with 1 pollock half.

5. Top each serving with half of the grapefruit, fennel, pepitas, and avocado.

PER SERVING Calories: 284; Total Fat: 7g; Protein: 25g; Carbohydrates: 11g; Sugars: 3g; Fiber: 5g; Sodium: 706mg

RECIPE TIP: *If you don't have Cajun seasoning, mix your own by combining 1 tablespoon of paprika, 1½ teaspoons of cayenne pepper, 1½ teaspoons of onion powder, ½ teaspoon of salt, ¼ teaspoon of white pepper, ¼ teaspoon of black pepper, ⅛ teaspoon of thyme, ⅛ teaspoon of dried basil, and ⅛ teaspoon of oregano.*

Five-Spice Tilapia

DAIRY-FREE • QUICK & EASY
PREP TIME: 15 MINUTES • COOK TIME: 5 MINUTES

Chinese five-spice powder adds a deliciously warm, spicy-sweet taste, and pleasant aroma to this simple and nutritious dish. Tilapia and crunchy sugar snap peas are cooked in a thick sauce that only takes minutes to prepare. Tilapia is one of the most popular fish consumed in the United States due to its good taste and relatively low cost. Tilapia is a flaky, white-meat fish that cooks up nicely however you choose to prepare it. Low in calories and high in heart-healthy omega-3 fats, protein, vitamins, and minerals, tilapia doesn't contain any carbohydrates. Whip up a side of Asian slaw by combining finely shredded napa cabbage, scallions, shredded carrots, and cilantro leaves.

8 ounces tilapia fillets

½ teaspoon Chinese five-spice powder

2 tablespoons reduced-sodium soy sauce

1 tablespoon granulated stevia

2 teaspoons extra-virgin olive oil

2 cups sugar snap peas

2 scallions, thinly sliced

1. Sprinkle both sides of the fillets with the Chinese five-spice powder.

2. In a small bowl, stir together the soy sauce and stevia. Set aside.

3. In a large nonstick skillet set over medium-high heat, heat the olive oil.

4. Add the tilapia. Cook for about 2 minutes, or until the outer edges are opaque. Reduce the heat to medium. Turn the fish over. Stir the soy mixture and pour into the skillet.

5. Add the sugar snap peas. Bring the sauce to a boil. Cook for about 2 minutes, or until the fish is cooked through, the sauce thickens, and the peas are bright green.

6. Add scallions. Remove from the heat.

7. Serve the fish and the sugar snap peas drizzled with the pan sauce.

PER SERVING Calories: 202; Total Fat: 7g; Protein: 26g; Carbohydrates: 7g; Sugars: 3g; Fiber: 0g; Sodium: 619mg

INGREDIENT TIP: *The soy sauce in this recipe can be replaced by Bragg Liquid Aminos, a gluten-free, non-GMO (genetically modified organism) lower-sodium seasoning. Bragg can be found in the vinegar and oil aisle in larger supermarkets. There is also a source link in the resources section.*

Fish Tacos

DAIRY-FREE • QUICK & EASY
PREP TIME: 10 MINUTES • COOK TIME: 10 MINUTES

Quick-cooking fish makes for a light and flavorful taco filling that's perfect for busy weeknights. This recipe uses tilapia fillets and replaces a higher-calorie beer batter with one using finely ground flaxseed meal and an egg wash. Flaxseed is rich in omega-3 fatty acids, fiber, and protein and the light, nutty flavor complements pan-seared food. A quick and easy-to-prepare homemade salsa tops this tasty and nutritious dish. Serve with a green salad and a side of steamed broccoli.

For the salsa

2 large tomatoes, diced

¼ cup diced red onion

2 to 3 tablespoons freshly
  squeezed lime juice

¼ teaspoon salt

⅛ teaspoon freshly ground
  black pepper

½ avocado, diced

¼ cup chopped fresh cilantro

For the tacos

1 large egg

3 tablespoons finely ground
  flaxseed meal

⅛ teaspoon ground cumin

⅛ teaspoon salt

⅛ teaspoon cayenne pepper
  (optional)

8 ounces tilapia fillet, sliced
  crosswise into 1-inch-
  wide strips

2 teaspoons extra-virgin
  olive oil

4 (6-inch) corn tortillas,
  warmed

To make the salsa

1. In a medium bowl, stir together the tomato, onion, lime juice, salt, and pepper.

2. Stir in the avocado and cilantro. Set aside.

To make the tacos

1. In a large bowl, whisk the egg until frothy.

2. Add the flaxseed meal, cumin, salt, and cayenne pepper (if using). Mix to create a batter.

3. In a large nonstick skillet set over medium-high heat, heat the olive oil.

4. Coat the tilapia pieces in the batter, letting the excess batter drip back into the bowl. Add the tilapia to the skillet. Cook for 2 to 4 minutes per side, or until crispy and golden.

5. Serve the fish with the warmed corn tortillas and salsa.

PER SERVING Calories: 431; Total Fat: 20g; Protein: 30g; Carbohydrates: 28g; Sugars: 1g; Fiber: 8g; Sodium: 163mg

INGREDIENT TIP: *Whole flaxseeds have an indigestible coating, so purchase them in finely ground meal form or grind whole seeds yourself in a clean coffee grinder. Grinding your own flaxseed meal lets you control the texture to your preference—a crunchy, grainy coating, or a finer flour-like finish.*

Sesame-Crusted Halibut

DAIRY-FREE
PREP TIME: 5 MINUTES, PLUS 15 MINUTES CHILLING TIME • COOK TIME: 15 MINUTES

Sesame seeds, marjoram, and basil form a crust that gives this dish its distinctive finish. Quickly roasting the fish at high heat keeps it moist and succulent so it melts in your mouth. Halibut is very low in calories and just one serving can help you meet more than 90 percent of the recommended daily amount of vitamin D, which is tough to get through diet alone. Sesame seeds give this dish even more bone-building power as they are a great source of phosphorus and calcium. Serve with a side of roasted vegetables and winter squash and a fresh green salad.

1 tablespoon freshly squeezed lemon juice

1 tablespoon extra-virgin olive oil

1 garlic clove, minced

Freshly ground black pepper, to season

1 (8-ounce) halibut fillet, halved

2 tablespoons sesame seeds, toasted

1 teaspoon dried basil

1 teaspoon dried marjoram

½ cup minced chives

⅛ teaspoon salt

2 lemon wedges

1. Preheat the oven to 450°F.

2. Line a baking sheet with aluminum foil.

3. In a shallow glass dish, mix together the lemon juice, olive oil, and garlic. Season with pepper.

4. Add the halibut and turn to coat. Cover and refrigerate for 15 minutes.

5. In a small bowl, combine the sesame seeds, basil, marjoram, and chives.

6. Remove the fish from the refrigerator. Sprinkle with the salt. Coat evenly with the sesame seed mixture, covering the sides as well as the top.

7. Transfer the fish to the prepared baking sheet. Place the sheet in the preheated oven. Roast for 10 to 14 minutes, or until just cooked through.

8. Garnish each serving with 1 lemon wedge.

PER SERVING Calories: 202; Total Fat: 11g; Protein: 24g; Carbohydrates: 2g; Sugars: 0g; Fiber: 1g; Sodium: 75mg

TOSS IT TOGETHER TIP: *To toast sesame seeds, place them in a small dry skillet and cook over medium-low heat for 2 to 4 minutes, stirring constantly, until fragrant and lightly browned. Top steamed or roasted vegetables with them, toss on salads, mix into hot cereal, and sprinkle them on pancakes.*

Greek Scampi

PREP TIME: 10 MINUTES • COOK TIME: 5 MINUTES

This Greek version of a classic shrimp dish is especially easy to prepare and superbly flavored. Nonfat ricotta cheese replaces the feta cheese to provide a dish lighter in salt, with less saturated fat. Ricotta cheese is a bit sweeter than feta, but its crumbly texture can serve the same purpose. Decorate with lemon wedges and serve with a side of steamed broccoli or asparagus.

2 garlic cloves, minced

2 tablespoons extra-virgin olive oil

½ pound shrimp, peeled, deveined, and thoroughly rinsed

1 cup diced tomatoes

½ cup nonfat ricotta cheese

6 Kalamata olives

Juice of ½ lemon

2 teaspoons chopped fresh dill, or ¾ teaspoon dried

Dash salt

Dash freshly ground black pepper

Lemon wedges, for garnish

1. In a large skillet set over medium heat, sauté the garlic in the olive oil for 30 seconds.

2. Add the shrimp. Cook for 1 minute.

3. Add the tomatoes, ricotta cheese, olives, lemon juice, and dill. Reduce the heat to low. Simmer for 5 to 10 minutes, stirring so the shrimp cook on both sides. When the shrimp are pink and the tomatoes and ricotta have made a sauce, the dish is ready.

4. Sprinkle with salt and pepper.

5. Serve immediately, garnished with lemon wedges.

PER SERVING Calories: 350; Total Fat: 20g; Protein: 30g; Carbohydrates: 11g; Sugars: 6g; Fiber: 1g; Sodium: 558mg

TOSS IT TOGETHER TIP: *Use ricotta cheese to make summer squash and ricotta "sandwiches." Simply grill slices of summer squash and spread with ricotta cheese. Place one slice on top of another to make a high-protein vegetable hors d'oeuvre or light lunch.*

Caribbean Haddock in a Packet

DAIRY-FREE • QUICK & EASY
PREP TIME: 10 MINUTES • COOK TIME: 20 MINUTES

While fancy in appearance, cooking fish in foil packets locks in moisture and flavor, making it a foolproof way to get tender, delicious results. Simply pile vegetables and fish on a foil square, seal, and bake. The contents will steam and the flavors will blend. This Caribbean-inspired recipe uses haddock, angel hair coleslaw, fresh lime juice, and cilantro for a fish dish with a kick. Haddock is super-low in calories, and high in protein and beneficial omega-3 fatty acids, making it a great choice to include in your diet on a regular basis.

1 tablespoon extra-virgin olive oil, divided

1 cup angel hair coleslaw, divided

1 (8-ounce) haddock fillet, halved and rinsed

1 small tomato, thinly sliced

1 small red bell pepper, thinly sliced

½ cup chopped fresh chives

2 tablespoons chopped fresh cilantro

Juice of 1 lime

4 dashes hot pepper sauce

Dash salt

Dash freshly ground black pepper

1. Preheat the oven to 450°F.

2. Fold 2 (12-by-24-inch) aluminum foil sheets in half widthwise into 2 (12-by-12-inch) squares.

3. In the center of each foil square, brush ½ teaspoon of olive oil.

4. Place ½ cup of coleslaw in each square.

5. Top each with 1 piece of haddock.

6. Add half of the tomato slices and half of the red bell pepper slices atop each fillet.

7. Sprinkle each with 1 of the remaining 2 teaspoons of olive oil, ¼ cup of chives, 1 tablespoon of cilantro, half of the lime juice, and 2 dashes of hot pepper sauce. Season with salt and pepper.

8. Fold and seal the foil into airtight packets. Place the packets in a baking dish and into the preheated oven. Bake for 20 minutes.

9. Carefully avoiding the steam that will be released, open a packet and check that the fish is cooked. It should be opaque and flake easily. To test for doneness, poke the tines of a fork into the thickest portion of the fish at a 45-degree angle. Gently twist the fork and pull up some of the fish. If the fish resists flaking, return it to the oven for another 2 minutes then test again. Fish cooks very quickly, so be careful not to overcook it.

10. Divide the fish, vegetables, and juices between 2 serving plates.

PER SERVING Calories: 227; Total Fat: 15g; Protein: 21g; Carbohydrates: 6g; Sugars: 4g; Fiber: 2g; Sodium: 117mg

TOSS IT TOGETHER TIP: *Serve this dish with baked or mashed sweet potatoes and a large green salad. For lower-carb mashed sweet potatoes, mash one small cooked sweet potato with 1 cup of cooked cauliflower, 1 to 2 tablespoons of nonfat Greek yogurt, 1 teaspoon of extra-virgin olive oil, and season with salt and pepper.*

Asian Salmon in a Packet

DAIRY-FREE • QUICK & EASY
PREP TIME: 10 MINUTES • COOK TIME: 20 MINUTES

Sesame oil, with its unique taste and aroma, creates a smooth and silky Asian sauce with just the right amount of garlic and ginger to make this dish melt in your mouth. Moist, flaky, juicy, and flavorful, the salmon is cooked in foil packets with rich-tasting shiitake mushrooms, high-fiber brown rice, and bok choy. Your taste buds won't believe how much flavor is packed into each delicious bite.

For the sauce

1 tablespoon extra-virgin olive oil, divided

1 teaspoon grated fresh ginger

1 garlic clove, minced

2 tablespoons low-sodium soy sauce

2 teaspoons dark sesame oil

For the salmon packets

1 teaspoon extra-virgin olive oil, divided

1 cup cooked brown rice, divided

2 cups coarsely chopped bok choy, divided

1 small red bell pepper, sliced, divided

½ cup sliced shiitake mushrooms, divided

2 (6-ounce) salmon steaks, rinsed

2 scallions, chopped, divided

To make the sauce

In a small bowl, whisk together the olive oil, ginger, garlic, soy sauce, and sesame oil. Set aside.

To make the salmon packets

1. Preheat the oven to 450°F.

2. Fold 2 (12-by-24-inch) aluminum foil sheets in half widthwise into 2 (12-by-12-inch) squares.

3. Brush ½ teaspoon of the olive oil in the center of each foil square.

4. Spread ½ cup of the rice in the center of each square.

5. Over the rice in each packet, layer 1 cup of bok choy, half of the red bell pepper slices, ¼ cup of mushrooms, 1 salmon steak, and half of the scallions.

6. Pour half of the sauce over each.

7. Fold and seal the foil into airtight packets. Place the packets in a baking dish and into the preheated oven. Bake for 20 minutes.

8. Carefully avoiding the steam that will be released, open a packet and check that the fish is cooked. It should be opaque and flake easily. To test for doneness, poke the tines of a fork into the thickest portion of the fish at a 45-degree angle. Gently twist the fork and pull up some of the fish. If the fish resists flaking, return it to the oven for another 2 minutes then test again. Fish cooks very quickly, so be careful not to overcook it.

9. Transfer the contents of the packets to serving plates or bowls.

10. Enjoy!

PER SERVING Calories: 426; Total Fat: 17g; Protein: 33g; Carbohydrates: 35g; Sugars: 4g; Fiber: 5g; Sodium: 711mg

RECIPE TIP: *Boost the vegetables by adding your favorites. Julienned daikon radish would make a flavorful addition. Daikon radishes are staples in Asian cuisine, and the name "daikon" is actually Japanese for "big root." Daikon has a mild taste and is very low in calories and high in fiber, vitamin C, and potassium. Slices make a nice crunchy addition to a salad or sandwich.*

Tarragon Cod in a Packet

DAIRY-FREE • QUICK & EASY

PREP TIME: 10 MINUTES • COOK TIME: 20 MINUTES

A popular and versatile herb, tarragon lends its unique mix of sweet aniseed-like and mild vanilla-like flavor to this moist and flaky cod dish. Steamed with a Mediterranean mix of vegetables, including zucchini, mushrooms, artichoke hearts, and black olives, this low-calorie dish is perfect on its own, with a large salad, or with a side of baked sweet potatoes.

1 tablespoon extra-virgin olive oil, divided

1 small zucchini, thinly sliced

1 cup sliced fresh mushrooms

2 (6-ounce) cod fillets, rinsed

½ red onion, thinly sliced

Juice of 1 lemon

¼ cup low-sodium vegetable broth

1 teaspoon dried tarragon

Dash salt

Dash freshly ground black pepper

1 (6.5-ounce) jar marinated quartered artichoke hearts, drained

6 black olives, halved and pitted

1. Preheat the oven to 450°F.

2. Fold 2 (12-by-24-inch) aluminum foil sheets in half widthwise into 2 (12-by-12-inch) squares.

3. Brush ½ teaspoon of olive oil in the center of each foil square.

4. In the middle of each square, layer, in this order, half of the zucchini slices, ½ cup of mushrooms, 1 cod fillet, and half of the onion slices.

5. Sprinkle each packet with 1 of the remaining 2 teaspoons of olive oil, half of the lemon juice, 2 tablespoons of vegetable broth, and ½ teaspoon of tarragon. Season with salt and pepper.

6. Top with half of the artichokes and 6 black olive halves.

7. Fold and seal the foil into airtight packets. Place the packets in a baking dish and into the preheated oven. Bake for 20 minutes.

8. Carefully avoiding the steam that will be released, open a packet and check that the fish is cooked. It should be opaque and flake easily. To test for doneness, poke the tines of a fork into the thickest portion of the fish at a 45-degree angle. Gently twist the fork and pull up some of the fish. If the fish resists flaking, return it to the oven for another 2 minutes then test again. Fish cooks very quickly, so be careful not to overcook it.

9. With a spatula, lift the fish and vegetables onto individual serving plates. Pour any liquid left in the foil over each serving.

10. Enjoy!

PER SERVING Calories: 316; Total Fat: 16g; Protein: 27g; Carbohydrates: 15g; Sugars: 6g; Fiber: 6g; Sodium: 1501mg

RECIPE TIP: *Side dishes that would complement this meal nicely include cauliflower "mashed potatoes," roasted peppers and eggplant, or a grain such as quinoa mixed with sun dried tomatoes. You could also serve the fish on mixed salad greens topped with a few slices of fresh tomato. If you don't have tarragon, try fresh or dried marjoram or basil instead.*

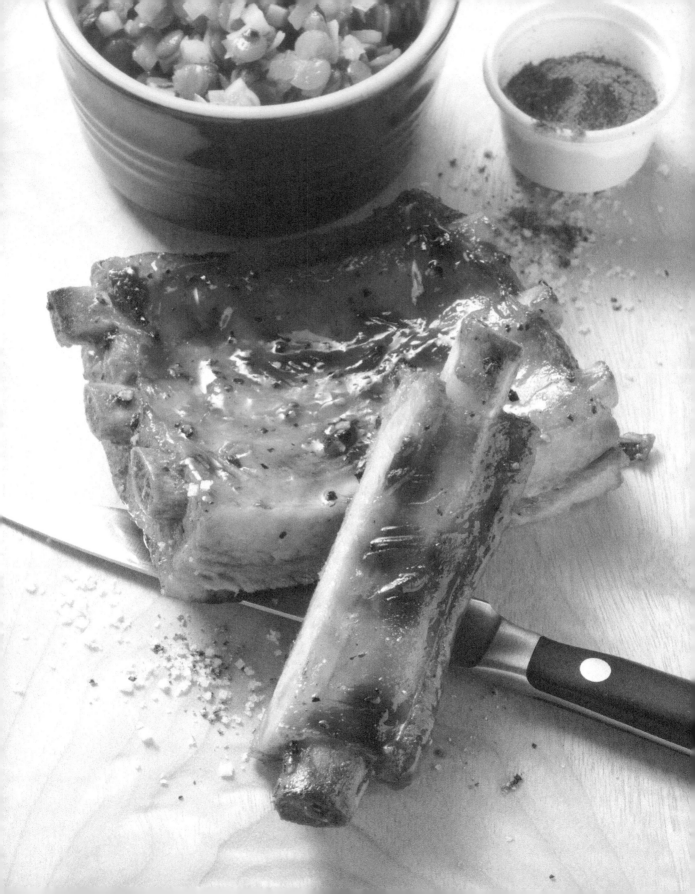

CHAPTER

9

Pork & Beef Entrées

Gingered-Pork Stir-Fry

DAIRY-FREE • QUICK & EASY
PREP TIME: 10 MINUTES • COOK TIME: 20 MINUTES

Why order Chinese take-out when it's so fun to make it yourself? This tasty recipe is lower in salt and unhealthy fat than most take-out meals, plus you can add your favorite vegetables or use whatever you have on hand. Economical, and much better for your health and waistline, this quick-and-easy pork stir-fry uses a simple yet delicious sauce to coat the meat and vegetables. Finished with crunchy cashews for additional heart-healthy fats, this dish comes together quickly, but tastes like you fussed.

2 tablespoons extra-virgin olive oil

2 garlic cloves, minced

1 (½-inch) piece fresh ginger, peeled, thinly sliced

¼ pound lean pork, thinly sliced

2 teaspoons low-sodium soy sauce

1 teaspoon granulated stevia

1 teaspoon sesame oil

1 cup snow peas

1 medium red bell pepper, sliced

6 whole fresh mushrooms, sliced

2 scallions, chopped

1 tablespoon Chinese rice wine

2 tablespoons chopped cashews, divided

1. In a large skillet or wok set over medium-high heat, heat the olive oil.

2. Add the garlic and ginger. Sauté for 1 to 2 minutes, or until fragrant.

3. Add the pork, soy sauce, and stevia. Cook for 10 minutes, stirring occasionally.

4. Stir in the sesame oil, snow peas, bell pepper, mushrooms, scallions, and rice wine. Reduce the heat to low. Simmer for 4 to 8 minutes, or until the pork is tender.

5. Divide between 2 serving plates, sprinkle each serving with 1 tablespoon of cashews and enjoy!

PER SERVING Calories: 426; Total Fat: 28g; Protein: 30g; Carbohydrates: 15g; Sugars: 4g; Fiber 3g; Sodium: 308mg

INGREDIENT TIP: *When buying fresh ginger, it should feel rock hard and the tan skin should look smooth and taut. Any root with wrinkled-looking skin should be avoided. It's best to buy a small amount at a time and store it in a plastic bag in the refrigerator's vegetable crisper. A good alternative to fresh ginger is finely grated or minced jarred ginger. Freshly grated ginger and jarred ginger are interchangeable in recipes. Depending on how often you make recipes calling for ginger, jarred may be the best choice for you.*

Pork and Cabbage Skillet

DAIRY-FREE

PREP TIME: 15 MINUTES • COOK TIME: 1 HOUR, 30 MINUTES

Is there a more perfect combination than pork, cabbage, and apples? Usually the cabbage comes in the form of sauerkraut, but it is just as easily sautéed with some onions and seasonings. Add a few crisp, tart apples for a sweet and sour punch and you have a healthy, satisfying meal—perfect for a chilly winter night. Serve with a green salad, or pair with Cauliflower "Mashed Potatoes" (page 176) and roasted asparagus for a fabulous gourmet-like meal.

2 tablespoons extra-virgin olive oil

2 (4-ounce) pork chops

½ medium head cabbage, quartered

2 onions, each quartered

1 tart apple, peeled, cored, and chopped

2½ cups water, divided

2 garlic cloves, crushed

2 teaspoons Worcestershire sauce

½ teaspoon salt

½ teaspoon freshly ground black pepper

2 tablespoons coconut flour

1. In a large skillet set over medium-high heat, heat the olive oil.

2. Add the pork chops. Cook for about 10 minutes per side, or until well-browned on each side.

3. Add the cabbage, onions, apple, 2 cups of water, garlic, Worcestershire sauce, salt, and pepper. Bring to a boil. Reduce the heat to medium-low. Cover and simmer for 45 minutes to 1 hour, or until the pork chops are completely tender.

4. Transfer the pork and vegetable mixture to a serving platter, leaving as much liquid in the skillet as possible. Return the skillet to the heat.

5. In a small bowl, whisk together the remaining ½ cup of water and the coconut flour.

6. Raise the heat under the skillet to medium-high. Pour the coconut flour mixture into the liquid remaining in the skillet. Cook for 1 to 2 minutes, stirring constantly, until the gravy thickens and begins to boil. Reduce the heat to low. Simmer for 5 minutes more.

7. Pour the gravy over the pork and vegetable mixture.

8. Serve immediately.

PER SERVING Calories: 448; Total Fat: 25g; Protein: 30g; Carbohydrates: 38g; Sugars: 13g; Fiber: 16g; Sodium: 390mg

Pork Tacos

DAIRY-FREE

PREP TIME: 15 MINUTES, PLUS 1 HOUR MARINATING TIME • COOK TIME: 10 MINUTES

This delicious recipe takes advantage of Mexico's gift to high-flavor cooking: chipotle peppers in adobo sauce. Typically sold in 7-ounce cans in the international foods section of many supermarkets, these peppers pack in gobs of smoky, chocolatey, slightly sweet, piquant flavor. Chipotles are just jalapeño peppers that have been dried and smoked. They are most often packed in adobo sauce, which is a smooth tomato-vinegar blend spiked with garlic, onion, and various spices. Flavorful and nutritious, these pork tacos offer an authentic taste of Mexico.

8 ounces boneless skinless pork tenderloin, thinly sliced, ¼-inch thick, across the grain

Pinch salt

⅓ cup ancho chile sauce

2 tablespoons chipotle purée (see Recipe Tip)

¼ cup freshly squeezed lime juice

2 (6-inch) soft low-carb corn tortillas, such as La Tortilla

4 tablespoons diced tomatoes, divided

1 cup shredded lettuce, divided

½ avocado, sliced

4 tablespoons salsa, divided

1. Sprinkle the pork slices with salt. Set aside.

2. In a small bowl, stir together the ancho chile sauce, chipotle purée, and lime juice. Reserve 3 tablespoons of the marinade. Set aside.

3. In a large sealable plastic bag, add the pork. Pour the remaining marinade over it. Seal the bag, removing as much air as possible. Marinate the meat for 20 minutes to 1 hour at room temperature, or refrigerate for several hours. Turn the meat twice while it marinates.

4. Place a small nonstick skillet over medium heat. Have a large piece of aluminum foil nearby.

5. Working with one tortilla at a time, heat both sides in the skillet until they puff slightly. As they are done, stack the tortillas on the foil. When they are all heated, wrap the tortillas in the foil.

6. Preheat the broiler.

7. Adjust the rack so it is 4 inches from the heating element.

8. Remove the pork slices from the marinade. Discard the marinade. Place the pork on a rack set over a sheet pan.

9. Place the pan in the oven. Broil for 3 to 4 minutes, or until the edges of the pork begin to brown. Remove from the oven. Turn and brush the pork with the reserved marinade. Broil the second side for 3 minutes, or until the pork is just barely pink inside.

10. Place the foil packet with the tortillas in the oven to warm while the pork finishes cooking.

11. To serve, pile each tortilla with a few slices of pork. Top each with about 2 tablespoons of diced tomato, ½ cup of shredded lettuce, half of the avocado slices, and about 2 tablespoons of salsa.

PER SERVING Calories: 392; Total Fat: 13g; Protein: 31g, Carbohydrates: 38g; Sugars: 16g; Fiber: 5g; Sodium: 1414mg

RECIPE TIP: *To make the chipotle purée, empty a can of chipotle chiles in adobo sauce into a small food processor or food chopper. Process into a smooth purée. It will keep for several weeks in the refrigerator, or freeze any leftovers.*

Grilled Pork Loin Chops

DAIRY-FREE

PREP TIME: 15 MINUTES, PLUS 8 HOURS MARINATING TIME • COOK TIME: 30 MINUTES

A mix of Asian ingredients gives these grilled chops lots of unique flavor. They can be broiled if you don't have a grill handy. If the chops are thick enough, they can be cut into kebab-size pieces, marinated in the refrigerator, and put on skewers with veggies of your choice. Steamed bok choy makes a great side. If it suits your taste, increase the amount of cinnamon, which research has shown to slow the rate at which the stomach empties after a meal—a plus for controlling blood-sugar levels.

2 garlic cloves, minced

3 tablespoons Worcestershire sauce

2 tablespoons water

1 tablespoon low-sodium soy sauce

2 teaspoons tomato paste

1 teaspoon granulated stevia

½ teaspoon ground ginger

½ teaspoon onion powder

¼ teaspoon cinnamon

⅛ teaspoon cayenne pepper

2 (6-ounce) thick-cut boneless pork loin chops

Olive oil, for greasing the grill

1. In a small bowl, mix together the garlic, Worcestershire sauce, water, soy sauce, tomato paste, stevia, ginger, onion powder, cinnamon, and cayenne pepper. Pour half of the marinade into a large plastic sealable bag. Cover and refrigerate the remaining marinade.

2. Add the pork chops to the bag and seal. Refrigerate for 4 to 8 hours, turning occasionally.

3. Preheat the grill to medium.

4. With the olive oil, lightly oil the grill grate.

5. Remove the pork chops from the bag. Discard the marinade in the bag.

6. Place the chops on the preheated grill, basting with the remaining reserved half of the marinade. Grill for 8 to 12 minutes per side, or until the meat is browned, no longer pink inside, and an instant-read thermometer inserted into the thickest part of the chop reads at least 145°F.

7. In a saucepan set over medium heat, pour any remaining reserved marinade. Bring to a boil. Reduce the heat to low. Simmer for about 5 minutes, stirring constantly, until slightly thickened.

8. To serve, plate the chops and spoon the sauce over.

PER SERVING Calories: 286; Total Fat: 13g; Protein: 36g; Carbohydrates: 8g; Sugars: 5g; Fiber: 0g; Sodium: 1015mg

RECIPE TIP: *If you don't have Worcestershire sauce, substitute Teriyaki Sauce (page 192) for equally great results. Stevia is an excellent replacement for sugar in cooking and baking. It not only sweetens foods, but also enhances the flavor. Stevia works especially well in sauces and dressings.*

Chinese Spareribs

DAIRY-FREE
PREP TIME: 10 MINUTES, PLUS 2 HOURS MARINATING TIME • COOK TIME: 40 MINUTES

The distinctive flavor of this dish comes from the hoisin sauce, sesame oil, and Chinese five-spice powder. If you want your ribs to have a deeper color, add some beet root powder or fermented red bean curd. Many Chinese restaurants use spareribs that are chopped into 3- to 4-inch riblets. Ask your butcher to do this, or make them whole. Enjoy this authentic-tasting Chinese meal with a simple side of stir-fried eggplant and bok choy.

2 tablespoons hoisin sauce

2 tablespoons tomato paste

2 tablespoons water

1 tablespoon rice vinegar

2 teaspoons sesame oil

2 teaspoons low-sodium soy sauce

2 teaspoons Chinese five-spice powder

2 garlic cloves, minced

1 teaspoon freshly squeezed lemon juice

1 teaspoon grated fresh ginger

½ teaspoon granulated stevia

1 pound pork spareribs

1. In a shallow glass dish, mix together the hoisin sauce, tomato paste, water, rice vinegar, sesame oil, soy sauce, Chinese five-spice powder, garlic, lemon juice, ginger, and stevia.

2. Add the ribs to the marinade. Turn to coat. Cover and refrigerate for 2 hours, or overnight.

3. Preheat the oven to 325°F.

4. Place a rack in the center of the oven.

5. Fill a broiler tray with enough water to cover the bottom. Place the grate over the tray. Arrange the ribs on the grate. Reserve the marinade.

6. Place the broiler pan in the preheated oven. Cook for 40 minutes, turning and brushing with the reserved marinade every 10 minutes.

7. Finish under the broiler for a crispier texture, if desired. Discard any remaining marinade.

8. Serve immediately with lots of napkins and enjoy!

PER SERVING Calories: 707; Total Fat: 61g; Protein: 34g; Carbohydrates: 8g; Sugars: 6g; Fiber: 1g; Sodium: 590mg

Open-Faced Pulled Pork

DAIRY-FREE

PREP TIME: 15 MINUTES • COOK TIME: 1 HOUR, 35 MINUTES

Pulled pork is made with a cooking method otherwise reserved for tough cuts of meat. Cooked slowly at a low temperature, the meat becomes tender enough to be "pulled," or easily torn into pieces. Pulled pork is usually served on a hamburger bun, but this recipe cuts the extra calories and carbs by using romaine lettuce leaves for an open-faced sandwich. Serve with a simple side of roasted vegetables, and enjoy the incredible flavor of this dish.

2 tablespoons hoisin sauce

2 tablespoons tomato paste

2 tablespoons rice vinegar

1 tablespoon minced fresh ginger

2 teaspoons minced garlic

1 teaspoon chile-garlic sauce

¾ pound pork shoulder, trimmed of any visible fat, cut into 2-inch-square cubes

4 large romaine lettuce leaves

1. Preheat the oven to 300°F.

2. In a medium ovenproof pot with a tight fitting lid, stir together the hoisin sauce, tomato paste, rice vinegar, ginger, garlic, and chile-garlic sauce.

3. Add the pork. Toss to coat.

4. Place the pot over medium heat. Bring to a simmer. Cover and carefully transfer the ovenproof pot to the preheated oven. Cook for 90 minutes.

5. Check the meat for doneness by inserting a fork into one of the chunks. If it goes in easily and the pork falls apart, the meat is done. If not, cook for another 30 minutes or so, until the meat passes the fork test.

6. Using a coarse strainer, strain the cooked pork into a fat separator. Shred the meat. Set aside. If you don't have a fat separator, remove the meat from the sauce and set aside. Let the sauce cool until any fat has risen to the top. With a spoon, remove as much fat as possible or use paper towels to blot it off.

(continued)

7. In a small saucepan set over high heat, pour the defatted sauce. Bring to a boil, stirring frequently to prevent scorching. Cook for 2 to 3 minutes, or until thickened.

8. Add the shredded meat. Toss to coat with the sauce. Cook for 1 minute to reheat the meat.

9. Spoon equal amounts of pork into the romaine lettuce leaves and enjoy!

PER SERVING Calories: 442; Total Fat: 25g; Protein: 42g; Carbohydrates: 9g; Sugars: 6g; Fiber: 4g; Sodium: 494mg

Sage-Parmesan Pork Chops

PREP TIME: 30 MINUTES • COOK TIME: 25 MINUTES

This easy pork chop dish has a crunchy and delicious coating made with soy Parmesan cheese, almond meal, flaxseed meal, sage, and lemon peel. These more nutritious substitutions for high-carb flour and bread crumbs make this a healthy dish that will become a fast favorite.

Extra-virgin olive oil cooking spray

2 tablespoons coconut flour

¼ teaspoon salt

Pinch freshly ground black pepper

¼ cup almond meal

½ cup finely ground flaxseed meal

½ cup soy Parmesan cheese

1½ teaspoons rubbed sage

½ teaspoon grated lemon zest

2 (4-ounce) boneless pork chops

1 large egg, lightly beaten

1 tablespoon extra-virgin olive oil

1. Preheat the oven to 425°F.

2. Lightly coat a medium baking dish with cooking spray.

3. In a shallow dish, mix together the coconut flour, salt, and pepper.

4. In a second shallow dish, stir together the almond meal, flaxseed meal, soy Parmesan cheese, sage, and lemon zest.

5. Gently press one pork chop into the coconut flour mixture to coat. Shake off any excess. Dip into the beaten egg. Press into the almond meal mixture. Gently toss between your hands so any coating that hasn't stuck can fall away. Place the coated chop on a plate. Repeat the process with the remaining pork chop and coating ingredients.

6. In a large skillet set over medium heat, heat the olive oil.

7. Add the coated chops. Cook for about 4 minutes per side, or until browned. Transfer to the prepared baking dish. Place the dish in the preheated oven. Bake for 10 to 15 minutes, or until the juices run clear and an instant-read thermometer inserted into the middle of the pork reads 160°F.

PER SERVING Calories: 618; Total Fat: 36g; Protein: 42g; Carbohydrates: 24g; Sugars: 2g; Fiber: 16g; Sodium: 1080mg

INGREDIENT TIP: *Galaxy Nutritional Foods sells a soy-based Parmesan cheese as well as a vegan Parmesan cheese. Products such as these have gone mainstream and should be easy to find. Check your grocer's produce section where the other vegetarian products like tofu are displayed.*

Meatloaf for Two

PREP TIME: 15 MINUTES • COOK TIME: 45 MINUTES

Meatloaf is definitely one meal you can have on a regular basis—with a few smart substitutions. The first should be for the bread crumbs, and this is easy to do. There are a number of good substitutes that provide the right consistency and taste, including almond meal and finely ground flaxseed. This recipe is just like Mom's but without the unhealthy ingredients. Plus, it sneaks in a few extra servings of vegetables for a beautiful result that is sure to please the palate. Serve with a simple salad and a side of steamed Brussels sprouts.

Extra-virgin olive oil cooking spray

1 large egg, beaten

1 cup frozen spinach

⅓ cup almond meal

¼ cup chopped onion

¼ cup nonfat milk

¼ teaspoon salt

¼ teaspoon dried sage

2 teaspoons extra-virgin olive oil, divided

Dash freshly ground black pepper

½ pound (96 percent) extra-lean ground beef

¼ cup tomato paste

1 tablespoon granulated stevia

¼ teaspoon Worcestershire sauce

1. Preheat the oven to 350°F.

2. Coat a shallow baking dish with cooking spray.

3. In a large bowl, combine the beaten egg, spinach, almond meal, onion, milk, salt, sage, 1 teaspoon of olive oil, and pepper.

4. Crumble the beef over the spinach mixture. Mix well to combine. Divide the meat mixture in half. Shape each half into a loaf. Place the loaves in the prepared dish.

5. In a small bowl, whisk together the tomato paste, stevia, Worcestershire sauce, and remaining 1 teaspoon of olive oil. Spoon half of the sauce over each meatloaf.

6. Place the dish in the preheated oven. Bake for 40 to 45 minutes, or until the meat is no longer pink and an instant-read thermometer inserted into the center reads 160°F.

7. Serve immediately and enjoy!

PER SERVING Calories: 396; Total Fat 22g; Protein 35g; Carbohydrates 16g; Sugars 7g; Fiber 7g; Sodium 477mg

RECIPE TIP: *Ketchup is a source of hidden sugar. A good substitute is plain tomato paste mixed with a dash of granulated stevia for a touch of sweetness, a dash of Worcestershire sauce, and a bit of extra-virgin olive oil to add richness. To make this dish even healthier, consider using a vegan Worcestershire sauce to eliminate anchovies and refined sugars. Try the Easy Ketchup (page 193), too!*

Herb-Marinated Tenderloins

DAIRY-FREE
PREP TIME: 10 MINUTES, PLUS 12 HOURS MARINATING TIME • COOK TIME: 20 MINUTES

Tenderloins are considered the gold standard of beef cuts. They are tender, rich, versatile, and easier to cook than you might think. The butcher will trim the tenderloin so only the most tender meat remains. Because this cut is so tender, it should be cooked using only dry-heat methods, such as broiling and grilling. This dish includes antioxidant-rich sweet potato and cherry tomatoes to complete the meal.

1 (8-ounce) beef tenderloin filet

6 fresh sage leaves

1 garlic clove, sliced into 6 pieces

4 fresh rosemary sprigs

Dash salt

Dash freshly ground black pepper

1 medium sweet potato

12 cherry tomatoes, chopped

1 tablespoon finely chopped fresh chives

2 teaspoons extra-virgin olive oil

4 cups baby spinach, divided

1. Cut 3 (2-inch-deep) slits in each side of the filet. Stuff 1 sage leave and 1 garlic slice into each slit. Wrap the rosemary sprigs around the filet. Season with salt and pepper. Refrigerate for 12 hours, or overnight, to allow the meat to absorb the seasoning flavors.

2. The next day, preheat the broiler to high.

3. Drain the steak. Place on an unheated rack in the broiler pan. Place the pan in the preheated oven. Broil the steak for 13 to 17 minutes for medium (160°F), 3 inches from the heat, turning once halfway through. Remove from the oven. Let the filet rest for 2 to 3 minutes before cutting in half. Tent with aluminum foil to keep warm.

4. While the filet cooks, poke the sweet potato all over with a fork. Microwave on high for about 6 minutes, or until soft. Thinly slice the cooked potato into rounds. Keep warm.

(continued)

5. In a small bowl, mix together the tomatoes, chives, and olive oil.

6. Place 2 cups of spinach on each serving plate. Arrange half of the sweet potato slices in a half-moon shape on each plate. Spoon half of the tomatoes over the sweet potatoes. Place 1 filet half in the center of each plate.

7. Enjoy!

PER SERVING Calories: 360; Total Fat: 14g; Protein: 40g; Carbohydrates: 41g; Sugars: 14g; Fiber: 10g; Sodium: 232mg

COOKING TIP: *To grill the beef on a charcoal grill, place the meat on an uncovered grill rack directly over medium coals. Grill to the desired doneness, turning once halfway through cooking. Allow 12 to 15 minutes for medium (160°F). If using a gas grill, preheat the grill, then reduce the heat to medium. Place the meat on the grill rack and cover. Cook to the desired doneness. Remove the steaks from the grill. Cover and let stand for 5 minutes.*

Italian Beef Kebabs

DAIRY-FREE

PREP TIME: 25 MINUTES, PLUS 1 HOUR MARINATING TIME • COOK TIME: 10 MINUTES

These robust beef kebabs pair marinated steak with a vegetable medley of summer squash, peppers, mushrooms, and onions to deliver a steak-house experience on a stick. The cut of meat provides the right balance between tenderness and flavor, and a delicious marinade of fresh herbs and balsamic vinegar gives these kebabs big flavor. A complete meal on a stick, customize this recipe with your favorite vegetables (more mushrooms, please!).

2 garlic cloves, finely chopped

¼ cup balsamic vinegar

¼ cup water

2 tablespoons extra-virgin olive oil

1 tablespoon chopped fresh oregano leaves, or 1 teaspoon dried

1½ teaspoons chopped fresh marjoram leaves, or ½ teaspoon dried

1 teaspoon granulated stevia

1 (¾-pound, 1-inch-thick) beef bone-in sirloin, or round steak, fat removed, cut into 1-inch pieces

1 medium yellow squash, sliced

1 medium green bell pepper, cut into 1-inch squares

6 whole fresh button mushrooms

1 small red onion, cut into 1-inch squares

1. In a medium glass bowl, mix together the garlic, balsamic vinegar, water, olive oil, oregano, marjoram, and stevia.

2. Add the beef. Stir until coated. Cover and refrigerate, stirring occasionally, for at least 1 hour but no longer than 12 hours.

3. Preheat the oven to broil.

4. Remove the beef from the marinade, reserving the marinade.

5. Using 10-inch metal skewers, thread on 1 piece of beef, 1 piece of yellow squash, 1 piece of bell pepper, 1 mushroom, and 1 piece of onion, leaving ½ inch of space between each piece. Repeat with the remaining ingredients until all are used. Brush the kebabs with the reserved marinade.

6. Place the kebabs on a rack in the broiler pan. Place the pan under the preheated broiler about 3 inches from the heat. Broil for 6 to 8 minutes for medium-rare to medium doneness, turning and brushing with the marinade after 3 minutes. Discard any remaining marinade.

7. Enjoy this delightful meal on a stick!

PER SERVING Calories: 548; Total Fat: 28g; Protein: 55g; Carbohydrates: 12g; Sugars: 5g; Fiber: 3g; Sodium: 115mg

TIP: *If you're tempted to save the extra marinade—don't. It needs to be discarded because it has been in contact with raw meat. Bacteria from the raw meat could transfer to the marinade.*

Beef Stew

DAIRY-FREE
PREP TIME: 30 MINUTES, PLUS 8 HOURS MARINATING TIME •
COOK TIME: 1 HOUR, 20 MINUTES

Hearty, tasty, chock-full of vegetables and protein, this beef stew is warmly comforting and certain to fill your belly. Beef, beets, Brussels sprouts, carrots, and portobello mushrooms are seasoned with thyme in this simple recipe. Perfect for any chilly day, this is comfort food at its best. It's so inexpensive to make, you won't believe the deeply satisfying flavors in each bowl. Serve with a green salad or on a bed of zucchini "noodles."

4 cups low-sodium beef broth, divided

3 tablespoons freshly squeezed lemon juice

2 teaspoons reduced-sodium soy sauce

2 teaspoons Worcestershire sauce

½ pound cubed beef stew meat

2 teaspoons extra-virgin olive oil

1 small onion, chopped

2 garlic cloves, minced

4 baby beets, tops removed, peeled, and cut into 1-inch cubes

1 cup chopped Brussels sprouts

2 medium carrots, sliced into 1-inch pieces

1 cup sliced baby portobello mushrooms

2 fresh thyme sprigs

⅛ teaspoon cayenne pepper

2 teaspoons cornstarch

1. In a large sealable plastic bag, combine 1 cup of beef broth, the lemon juice, soy sauce, and Worcestershire sauce. Add the beef. Seal the bag, turning to coat. Refrigerate for 8 hours, or overnight.

2. The next day, drain the beef and discard the marinade.

3. In a large saucepan set over medium heat, combine the olive oil and drained beef. Cook for 8 to 10 minutes, or until browned. Transfer the meat to a bowl and set aside.

4. To the same saucepan, add the onion. Sauté for 5 to 7 minutes, or until tender.

5. Add the garlic. Cook for 1 minute.

6. Add 2½ cups of beef broth. Return the meat to the pan. Increase the heat to high. Bring to a boil. Reduce the heat to low. Cover and simmer for 30 minutes.

7. Add the beets, Brussels sprouts, carrots, mushrooms, thyme, and cayenne pepper. Increase the heat to high. Return to a boil. Reduce the heat to low. Cover and simmer for 30 minutes, or until the vegetables and beef are tender. Remove and discard the thyme sprigs.

8. In a small bowl, whisk together the cornstarch and remaining ½ cup of beef broth until smooth. Gradually add to the stew, stirring to incorporate. Increase the heat to high. Bring to a boil again. Cook for 2 minutes, stirring, or until thickened.

PER SERVING Calories: 361; Total Fat: 11g; Protein: 35g; Carbohydrates: 31g; Sugars: 13g; Fiber: 7g; Sodium: 812mg

COOKING TIP: *Plan ahead and prepare this stew in a slow cooker. Slow cookers are inexpensive to buy, economical to use, and great for making the most of budget ingredients. They offer a healthier, low-fat method of cooking and require a minimal amount of effort. They come in different sizes, as well—mini crockpots are perfect for making steel-cut oats for two, while the larger size is best suited for meal-size recipes.*

Peppered Beef with Greens and Beans

DAIRY-FREE • QUICK & EASY
PREP TIME: 10 MINUTES • COOK TIME: 20 MINUTES

Some pairings work so well together that they span generations. In the world of food, there are few combinations as fabled as pepper and steak. Black pepper is often just an afterthought or supplementary seasoning, at best. In this dish, the beef and black pepper are the stars while the bell peppers, onions, greens, and beans help take some of the edge off the spicy pepper. Enjoy with a large green salad or over a bed of vegetable "noodles."

1 (½-pound, ½-inch-thick) boneless beef sirloin, halved

2 teaspoons coarsely ground black pepper, divided

¼ cup tomato sauce

2 tablespoons red wine vinegar

1 teaspoon dried basil

3 cups (1 bunch) chopped kale

1 cup chopped green beans

¾ cup chopped red bell pepper, or yellow bell pepper

¼ cup chopped onion

1. Rub each side of the steak halves with ½ teaspoon of coarsely ground pepper.

2. Heat a 10-inch nonstick skillet over medium heat. Add the beef. Cook for 8 to 12 minutes, turning once halfway through.

3. Add the tomato sauce, red wine vinegar, and basil. Stir to combine.

4. Add the kale, green beans, bell pepper, and onion. Stir to mix with the sauce. Reduce the heat to medium-low. Cook for about 5 minutes, uncovered, or until the vegetables are tender and beef is cooked medium doneness (160°F).

5. Serve immediately and enjoy!

PER SERVING Calories: 372; Total Fat: 17g; Protein: 35g; Carbohydrates: 22g; Sugars: 4g; Fiber: 6g; Sodium: 349mg

RECIPE TIP: *Instead of serving over high-carb pasta, try cooked spaghetti squash or vegetable noodles, like carrot noodles or zucchini noodles, made with a spiralizer or julienne peeler. Angel hair coleslaw can also be used as a pasta stand in. Simply combine the cabbage with the extra-virgin olive oil in a pan and cook until crisp-tender.*

Teriyaki Rib-Eye Steaks

DAIRY-FREE • QUICK & EASY
PREP TIME: 10 MINUTES • COOK TIME: 15 MINUTES

This recipe cuts prep time to a minimum using powdered onion, garlic, and ginger. The sauce is sweetened without honey or sugar, but instead includes granulated stevia, a natural plant-based chemical-free alternative. This delicious one-pot meal is loaded with several servings of vegetables along with the high-protein rib-eye steaks. For added crunch, top with chopped peanuts or cashews.

2 tablespoons water

1 tablespoon reduced-sodium soy sauce

1½ teaspoons Worcestershire sauce

1¼ teaspoons distilled white vinegar

1 teaspoon extra-virgin olive oil

½ teaspoon granulated stevia

½ teaspoon onion powder

¼ teaspoon garlic powder

⅛ teaspoon ground ginger

2 (6-ounce) lean beef rib-eye steaks

Extra-virgin olive oil cooking spray

2 cups sugar snap peas

1 cup sliced carrots

1 red bell pepper, sliced

1. In a large bowl, whisk together the water, soy sauce, Worcestershire sauce, white vinegar, olive oil, stevia, onion powder, garlic powder, and ginger.

2. With a fork, pierce the steaks several times. Add to the marinade. Let marinate in the refrigerator for at least 2 hours.

3. Spray a large skillet with cooking spray. Place it over medium heat.

4. Add the steaks. Cook for 7 minutes. Turn the steaks. Add the sugar snap peas, carrots, and bell pepper to the skillet. Cook for 7 minutes more, or until an instant-read thermometer inserted into the center of the steak reads 140°F.

5. Serve and savor!

PER SERVING Calories: 641; Total Fat: 40g; Protein: 48g; Carbohydrates: 23g; Sugars: 13g; Fiber: 4g; Sodium: 725mg

INGREDIENT TIP: *To lower the sodium even further, the low-sodium soy sauce can be replaced with Bragg Liquid Aminos, which is a gluten-free, soy-based seasoning sauce. Made from the building blocks of protein, liquid aminos usually contain only a small amount of naturally occurring sodium, far less than in regular soy sauce.*

Grilled Steak and Vegetables

DAIRY-FREE

PREP TIME: 15 MINUTES • COOK TIME: 25 MINUTES

This simple recipe features sirloin steaks grilled with an assortment of vegetables. Grilling cooks the meat to melt-in-your-mouth tenderness and imparts a rich, smoky taste to the vegetables. Fragrant herb basil, with its bright, pungent, peppery taste, seasons the vegetables. High in protein, with several servings of vegetables, this is a complete and satisfying meal that can be eaten on its own or with a fresh garden salad.

Extra-virgin olive oil cooking spray

2 (8-ounce) sirloin steaks

2 medium pear-shaped tomatoes, halved lengthwise

1 medium zucchini, cut into chunks

1 medium yellow squash, cut into chunks

1 bell pepper (any color), cut into 1-inch pieces

2 tablespoons extra-virgin olive oil, divided

1 garlic clove, minced

¼ cup fresh basil, plus fresh sprigs, for garnish

Pinch salt

Freshly ground black pepper, to season

1. Preheat the grill (charcoal or gas).

2. Lightly coat a grill rack with cooking spray.

3. Place the steaks on the grill rack, about 4 to 6 inches above the heat—whether a solid bed of medium-hot coals or gas. Cook for about 15 minutes, turning as needed, until evenly browned on the outside and an instant-read thermometer inserted in the center registers 145°F for medium-rare.

4. While the steaks cook, place the tomatoes, zucchini, yellow squash, and bell pepper on the grill. Brush lightly with 1 tablespoon of olive oil. Grill for about 3 minutes, or until the vegetables are browned on the bottom. Turn them over. Continue to cook for about 3 minutes more, or until soft.

5. In a medium skillet with a heatproof handle set over medium-high heat, stir together the remaining 1 tablespoon of olive oil, garlic, and basil.

6. Transfer the grilled vegetables to the skillet. Stir to combine. Reduce the heat to low.

7. Serve each steak accompanied by half of the vegetables. Season with salt and pepper. Garnish with the basil sprigs.

PER SERVING Calories: 441; Total Fat: 21g; Protein: 51g; Carbohydrates: 13g; Sugars: 8g; Fiber: 4g; Sodium: 137mg

Marjoram-Pepper Steaks

DAIRY-FREE • QUICK & EASY
PREP TIME: 5 MINUTES • COOK TIME: 8 MINUTES

Sweet marjoram and pepper create a flavorful coating for beef tenderloins. Black pepper was once so valued it was used as a currency and presented to the gods as a sacred offering. Today, a pinch is added to just about every recipe. Black pepper has components that stimulate the stomach to increase digestive juices, promoting intestinal health. Contrasted with the sweet flavor and pungent taste of marjoram, this easy steak dish works well with a side of garlic-roasted vegetables, Brussels sprouts, or a simple garden salad.

1 tablespoon freshly ground black pepper

¼ teaspoon dried marjoram

2 (6-ounce, 1-inch-thick) beef tenderloins

1 tablespoon extra-virgin olive oil

¼ cup low-sodium beef broth

Fresh marjoram sprigs, for garnish

1. In a large bowl, mix together the pepper and marjoram.

2. Add the steaks. Coat both sides with the spice mixture.

3. In a skillet set over medium-high heat, heat the olive oil.

4. Add the steaks. Cook for 5 to 7 minutes, or until an instant-read thermometer inserted in the center registers 160°F (for medium). Remove from the skillet. Cover to keep warm.

5. Add the broth to the skillet. Increase the heat to high. Bring to a boil, scraping any browned bits from the bottom. Boil for about 1 minute, or until the liquid is reduced by half.

6. Spoon the broth sauce over the steaks. Garnish with marjoram sprigs and serve immediately.

PER SERVING Calories: 398; Total Fat: 21g; Protein: 49g; Carbohydrates: 2g; Sugars: 0g; Fiber: 1g; Sodium: 119mg

RECIPE TIP: *Use brandy or dry red wine in place of the beef broth. However, contrary to popular belief, alcohol does not completely evaporate during cooking so there will be trace amounts in the dish. A compromise is a nonalcoholic red wine or grape, cranberry, or pomegranate juice. For a dash of sweetness, add some stevia.*

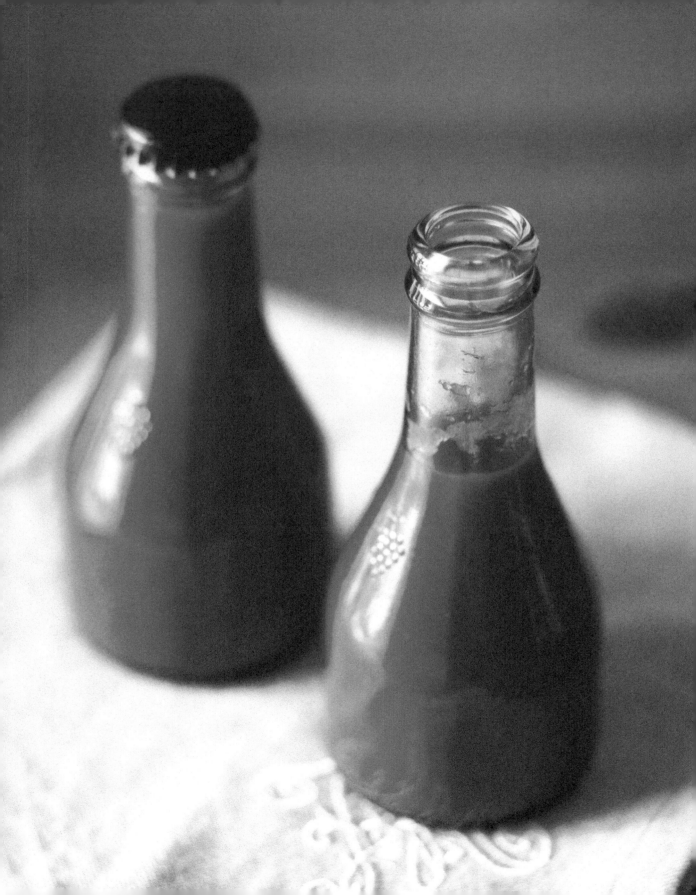

chapter 10

Sides & Staples

Cauliflower "Mashed Potatoes"

QUICK & EASY
PREP TIME: 5 MINUTES

Mashed potatoes are a classic any-meal side dish and a staple on most Thanksgivings tables. Unfortunately, the traditional ingredients—russet potatoes mashed with butter, cream, milk, and salt—result in a dish that's loaded in calories, carbs, saturated fat, and cholesterol. Yikes! Enter this creative recipe for faux mashed potatoes that tastes so close to the real deal you won't know the difference. Phytochemical- and vitamin C-rich cauliflower steps in for the potatoes, and nonfat Greek yogurt for the cream and butter. Finally, you can enjoy "mashed potatoes" and even indulge in a second helping or two.

2 cups cooked
    cauliflower florets
1 tablespoon plain nonfat
    Greek yogurt
½ teaspoon extra-virgin
    olive oil
Salt, to season
Freshly ground black pepper,
    to season

1. To a food processor, add the cauliflower, yogurt, and olive oil. Process until smooth.

2. Season with salt and pepper before serving.

PER SERVING Calories: 39; Total Fat: 1g; Protein: 2g; Carbohydrates: 4g; Sugars: 2g; Fiber: 0g; Sodium: 29mg

SERVING TIP: *Serve these "potatoes" with meatloaf, steak, pork chops, chicken breast, or as a side to veggie burgers. Top with chopped herbs and soy Parmesan cheese, or nonfat ricotta cheese. As your palate adjusts, try mashing other vegetables into the mix, like butternut squash for a touch of sweetness.*

Roasted Peppers and Eggplant

DAIRY-FREE • QUICK & EASY
PREP TIME: 5 MINUTES • COOK TIME: 20 MINUTES

If you think you don't like vegetables, roast them and try them again. Roasting vegetables gives off an irresistible aroma and produces a tantalizing taste that is hard to resist. As an added bonus, this cooking method helps make many of the nutrients in the vegetables more easily digestible, meaning your body absorbs more of the valuable vitamins and minerals they contain. Use whatever vegetables you have on hand and follow this same basic recipe.

Extra-virgin olive oil cooking spray

1 small eggplant, halved and sliced

1 red bell pepper, cut into thick strips

1 yellow bell pepper, cut into thick strips

1 red onion, sliced

2 garlic cloves, quartered

1 tablespoon extra-virgin olive oil

Salt, to season

Freshly ground black pepper, to season

½ cup chopped fresh basil

1. Preheat the oven to 350°F.

2. Coat a nonstick baking dish with cooking spray.

3. To the prepared dish, add the eggplant, red bell pepper, yellow bell pepper, onion, and garlic. Drizzle with the olive oil. Toss to coat well. Spray any uncoated surfaces with cooking spray.

4. Place the dish in the preheated oven. Bake for 20 minutes, turning once halfway through cooking.

5. Transfer the vegetables to a serving dish. Season with salt and pepper.

6. Garnish with the basil and serve.

PER SERVING Calories: 160; Total Fat: 7g; Protein: 4g; Carbohydrates: 23g; Sugars: 10g; Fiber: 10g; Sodium: 11mg

SERVING TIP: *This dish can be served with any lean meat, sautéed beans, scrambled eggs, veggie burgers, or as a topping for grains or spaghetti squash "noodles." Turn omelets into a gourmet meal by adding ½ to 1 cup of roasted vegetables to your eggs and top with ricotta cheese. Make a fast lunch wrap by serving roasted vegetables in lettuce leaves topped with beans or cheese.*

Sautéed Spinach with Parmesan and Almonds

PREP TIME: 5 MINUTES • COOK TIME: 5 MINUTES

If you aren't a fan of salads, try sautéing the greens. This quick and easy recipe is a simple sauté of prewashed bagged spinach with garlic and balsamic vinegar. Balsamic vinegar and its sweet, sour, woody taste goes nicely with a number of dishes, savory and sweet alike. Finished with vitamin E-rich almonds, this nutritious side dish is low in calories and sure to become a favorite. Serve with any type of meat, beans, or over grains.

2 teaspoons extra-virgin
   olive oil

2 tablespoons sliced almonds

2 garlic cloves, minced

2 (5-ounce) bags
   prewashed spinach

2 teaspoons balsamic vinegar

⅛ teaspoon salt

2 tablespoons soy
   Parmesan cheese

Freshly ground black pepper,
   to season

1. In a large nonstick skillet or Dutch oven set over medium-high heat, heat the olive oil.

2. Add the almonds and garlic. Cook for 30 seconds, stirring, or until fragrant.

3. Add the spinach. Cook for about 2 minutes, stirring, until just wilted. Remove the pan from the heat.

4. Stir in the balsamic vinegar and salt.

5. Sprinkle with the soy Parmesan cheese. Season with pepper and serve immediately.

PER SERVING Calories: 148; Total Fat: 9g; Protein: 8g; Carbohydrates: 8g; Sugars: 1g; Fiber: 3g; Sodium: 243mg

Braised Kale with Ginger and Sesame Seeds

DAIRY-FREE • QUICK & EASY
PREP TIME: 5 MINUTES • COOK TIME: 25 MINUTES

Kale is braised with pungent and spicy ginger and garnished with sesame seeds in this recipe. Because each food has a different array of phytochemicals, vitamins, and minerals, it is good for your health and your body to mix it up, eating different types of foods within the same food group. While all greens are nutritious, kale is higher in protein, calcium, and vitamins A, C, and K than most other greens. Because it is heavier and denser when cooked, it retains more texture than softer greens like spinach. For an added crunch and extra calcium, sesame seeds top off the finished dish.

¼ cup balsamic vinegar

1 garlic clove, minced

2 teaspoons chopped
     fresh ginger

6 cups (2 bunches) chopped
     kale, thoroughly washed
     and stemmed

¼ cup water, plus additional
     as needed

1 tablespoon sesame seeds

1. In a saucepan set over medium heat, whisk together the balsamic vinegar, garlic, and ginger. Cook for 5 minutes.

2. Add the kale. Stir to combine. Cook for 10 to 15 minutes, or until wilted.

3. Add the water. Cover and simmer for 2 minutes, adding more water as needed to keep the kale from sticking. Uncover and cook for 1 to 2 minutes more, or until any remaining liquid evaporates.

4. Sprinkle with the sesame seeds and serve.

PER SERVING Calories: 135; Total Fat: 5g; Protein: 7g; Carbohydrates: 20g; Sugars: 6g; Fiber: 4g; Sodium: 46mg

TOSS IT TOGETHER TIP: *Add leftover sesame seeds to hot cereals or baked goods, or use as a topping for salads, roasted vegetables, sautéed beans, and roasted meats. If you are short on time or concerned about spoilage, skip the fresh ginger and buy a jar of minced ginger. It keeps in the refrigerator and you'll have it on hand to add to your all of your favorite recipes.*

Green Beans with Red Peppers

DAIRY-FREE • QUICK & EASY
PREP TIME: 5 MINUTES • COOK TIME: 15 MINUTES

Tender, flexible green beans are a vegetarian's delight. Green beans, also known as string beans or snap beans, are fat free, very low in calories, and low in carbohydrates. Green beans have impressive amounts of antioxidants and even provide cardiovascular benefits. Rich in fiber, folate, and vitamins A and C, this recipe pairs this tasty bean with rich-tasting sun-dried tomatoes and red peppers for a delectable accompaniment to baked or grilled meats, or as a topping for grains.

8 ounces fresh green beans, broken into 2-inch pieces

6 sun-dried tomatoes (not packed in oil), halved

1 medium red bell pepper, cut into ¼-inch strips

1 teaspoon extra-virgin olive oil

Salt, to season

Freshly ground black pepper, to season

1. In a 1-quart saucepan set over high heat, add the green beans to 1 inch of water. Bring to a boil. Boil for 5 minutes, uncovered.

2. Add the sun-dried tomatoes. Cover and boil 5 to 7 minutes more, or until the beans are crisp-tender, and the tomatoes have softened. Drain. Transfer to a serving bowl.

3. Add the red bell pepper and olive oil. Season with salt and pepper. Toss to coat.

4. Serve warm.

PER SERVING Calories: 90; Total Fat: 2g; Protein: 4g; Carbohydrates: 16g; Sugars: 9g; Fiber: 5g; Sodium: 220mg

TOSS IT TOGETHER TIP: *Serve this dish with hummus for a healthy fast lunch or light supper. Try it topped with Parmesan cheese or nonfat ricotta cheese and fresh basil for a Mediterranean-inspired dish, or serve as a side for frittatas or other egg-based dishes.*

Broccoli with Pine Nuts

DAIRY-FREE • QUICK & EASY
PREP TIME: 10 MINUTES • COOK TIME: 5 MINUTES

This dish is a mix of broccoli florets and broccoli rabe (pronounced *rob*) sautéed simply with garlic. Broccoli rabe looks like broccoli with long, thin, leafy stalks topped with small florets, but is part of the turnip family. Sometimes referred to as rapini, this elegant and nutritious staple will be right at home in your kitchen. Topped with crunchy, buttery-tasting pine nuts and a squeeze of lemon, this dish is high in antioxidants, phytochemicals, vitamins A and C, and fiber.

1 bunch broccoli rabe

4 cups water

1 cup broccoli florets

1 tablespoon extra-virgin olive oil

2 medium garlic cloves, minced

1 tablespoon freshly squeezed lemon juice

Salt, to season

Freshly ground black pepper, to season

2 tablespoons pine nuts

1. Rinse the broccoli rabe well in cold water to remove any dirt particles. Tear into stalks. Set aside.

2. In a saucepan set over high heat, bring the water to a boil.

3. Place a colander in the sink. Add the broccoli rabe pieces and broccoli florets. Pour the boiling water over them to scald. Drain well. Set aside.

4. In a sauté pan or skillet set over medium heat, heat the olive oil.

5. Add the garlic. Sauté for 1 minute, or until browned.

6. Add the broccoli rabe and broccoli florets. Toss to coat with the garlic. Cook for about 3 minutes, or until heated through.

7. Drizzle the vegetables with the lemon juice. Season with salt and pepper.

8. Top with the pine nuts and serve.

PER SERVING Calories: 157; Total Fat: 14g; Protein: 4g; Carbohydrates: 6g; Sugars: 1g; Fiber: 1g; Sodium: 10mg

TOSS IT TOGETHER TIP: *Despite the name, pine nuts are not actually nuts but the seeds of the pine cone. They have been a popular source of nutrition since Paleolithic times and are used in pesto to add their distinct, delicious flavor and texture. Rich in heart-healthy fats, vitamins, and minerals, use any remaining pine nuts to make your own homemade pesto by processing with basil, garlic, and soy Parmesan cheese.*

Sweet-and-Sour Cabbage Slaw

DAIRY-FREE • QUICK & EASY
PREP TIME: 5 MINUTES

This simple sweet-and-sour slaw uses pre-sliced angel hair cabbage as a time saver, apple cider vinegar for a touch of sour flavor, a tart apple, and granulated stevia for a touch of sweetness. Sugar-free and high in cholesterol-lowering fiber, and vitamins A, C, and E, this dish works equally well accompanying a pork dish as it does one with Asian seasonings. To pair with an Asian dish, omit the apple and add grated fresh ginger.

2 tablespoons apple
  cider vinegar
1 tablespoon granulated stevia
2 cups angel hair cabbage
1 tart apple, cored and diced
½ cup shredded carrot
2 medium scallions, sliced
2 tablespoons sliced almonds

1. In a medium bowl, stir together the vinegar and stevia.

2. In a large bowl, mix together the cabbage, apple, carrot, and scallions.

3. Pour the sweetened vinegar over the vegetable mixture. Toss to combine.

4. Garnish with the sliced almonds and serve.

PER SERVING Calories: 100; Total Fat: 4g; Protein: 3g; Carbohydrates: 16g; Sugars: 9g; Fiber: 5g; Sodium: 59mg

INGREDIENT TIP: *To get the most nutrition from the foods you eat, leave the skin and peel of vegetables intact—they contain the fiber. Apple skins contain pectin, which is a type of soluble fiber known to reduce levels of LDL "bad" cholesterol. Wash thoroughly to remove any excess debris.*

Orange-Scented Asparagus with Sweet Red Peppers

DAIRY-FREE • QUICK & EASY
PREP TIME: 5 MINUTES • COOK TIME: 15 MINUTES

Spring is when asparagus is at its best—fresh, local, full of taste, and loaded with vitamins and minerals. Here, fresh asparagus is sautéed with red bell peppers, seasoned with orange zest, and then lightly browned under the broiler. This creative melding of flavors pairs well with a simple broiled fish or baked chicken. For added protein, sauté a few cubes of tofu with the red peppers.

⅓ pound fresh asparagus, trimmed

1 teaspoon extra-virgin olive oil mixed with 1 teaspoon warm water

1 red bell pepper, seeded and julienned

1 tablespoon grated orange zest

Salt, to season

Freshly ground black pepper, to season

1 teaspoon granulated stevia, divided

1. Preheat the broiler to high.

2. In a steamer or large pot of boiling water, cook the asparagus for about 7 minutes, or until barely tender. Drain. Set aside.

3. In a small skillet set over medium-high heat, heat the olive oil and water.

4. Add the bell pepper. Cook for about 5 minutes, stirring frequently, until slightly softened. Remove from the heat.

5. Stir in the orange zest. Season with salt and pepper.

6. Evenly divided the asparagus between 2 gratin dishes. Spoon half of the red bell pepper and sauce over each. Sprinkle each with ½ teaspoon of stevia. Place the dishes under the preheated broiler. Broil for 2 to 3 minutes, or until lightly browned.

7. Serve immediately.

PER SERVING Calories: 47; Total Fat: 2g; Protein: 1g; Carbohydrates: 5g; Sugars: 2g; Fiber: 2g; Sodium: 10mg

RECIPE TIP: *Au gratin dishes are typically used for broiling when the recipe calls for a browned or crisped topping. If you don't have an au gratin dish, use an ovenproof skillet or ramekin.*

INGREDIENT TIP: *Orange zest can be purchase in dried form, or simply grate the skin of a washed orange, and use the remaining fruit as a snack.*

Cheesy Broiled Tomatoes

QUICK & EASY

PREP TIME: 5 MINUTES • COOK TIME: 10 MINUTES

This quick and easy, cheesy broiled tomato dish features fresh tomatoes topped with high-protein nonfat ricotta cheese and fresh basil, and is cooked briefly under the broiler. A simple and uncomplicated recipe, these tomatoes make a great afternoon snack to hold you between lunch and dinner. They can also be a side to an egg dish, an accompaniment to a tuna salad wrap, or served with a piece of simply grilled fish or chicken. Vary the seasonings depending on your tastes.

2 large ripe tomatoes, halved widthwise

¼ cup nonfat ricotta cheese, divided

½ teaspoon dried basil, divided

Salt, to season

Freshly ground black pepper, to season

1. Preheat the broiler.

2. Top each tomato half with 1 tablespoon of ricotta cheese. Sprinkle with ⅛ teaspoon of basil. Season with salt and pepper.

3. On a broiler rack, place the tomatoes cut-side up. Place the rack into the preheated oven. Broil for 7 to 10 minutes.

4. Enjoy!

PER SERVING Calories: 53; Total Fat: 0g; Protein: 5g; Carbohydrates: 9g; Sugars: 6g; Fiber: 2g; Sodium: 75mg

INGREDIENT TIP: *Spices and herbs are an essential part of any pantry. While they won't spoil, they will lose their flavor over time. Check the use-by dates of any you have on hand, and replace those that have passed their expiration date. If you will only be using a small amount of a certain herb for a particular recipe, buy only the amount you need from the bulk bin of your local health food store.*

Zucchini Ribbons with Tarragon

QUICK & EASY
PREP TIME: 5 MINUTES • COOK TIME: 1 MINUTE

Zucchini ribbons, or "noodles," are seasoned here with the bittersweet flavor of tarragon. Ricotta cheese melts into the ribbons, which are tossed with pine nuts for a dish that is creamy, crunchy, flavorful, and, most importantly, healthy. Serve with egg dishes, meats, soups, stews, sautéed beans, or tofu. For even more anise flavor, add a dash of fennel seed.

1 zucchini, thinly sliced lengthwise into ribbons

1 tablespoon nonfat ricotta cheese

1 tablespoon pine nuts

1 tablespoon fresh tarragon

1½ teaspoons extra-virgin olive oil

½ to 1 teaspoon red pepper flakes

1. Bring a large pot of water to a boil.

2. Add the zucchini. Cook for 30 to 60 seconds, or until crisp-tender. Drain. Transfer the zucchini to a serving bowl.

3. Add the ricotta cheese, pine nuts, tarragon, olive oil, and red pepper flakes. Gently toss until the zucchini is coated.

4. Serve and enjoy!

PER SERVING Calories: 102; Total Fat: 7g; Protein: 4g; Carbohydrates: 7g; Sugars: 5g; Fiber: 2g; Sodium: 34mg

RECIPE TIP: *Consider buying an inexpensive spiralizer or julienne peeler for making vegetable ribbons. You can use an assortment of favorites, including carrots, yellow squash, butternut squash, beets, and other root vegetables like parsnips, turnips, and daikon radish. Use your imagination and try these nutritious ribbons anywhere you would normally use pasta.*

Italian-Style Spaghetti Squash

QUICK & EASY
PREP TIME: 10 MINUTES • COOK TIME: 15 MINUTES

Spaghetti squash is a yellow mild-flavored winter squash with an oblong shape. After cooking and running a fork through it, the flesh separates into spaghetti-like strands. It is the ideal substitute for pasta thanks to its low-carbohydrate and low-calorie counts. This recipe can be used as a side dish to meats or fish, or add ricotta cheese, sautéed tofu, or ground meat for a complete meal.

1 (1-pound) spaghetti squash, halved lengthwise and seeded

¼ cup water

3 teaspoons extra-virgin olive oil, divided, plus additional as needed

1 small red onion, sliced

1 small zucchini, cut into ½-inch slices

1 medium tomato, diced

¼ teaspoon salt

1 teaspoon dried oregano

1 teaspoon dried basil

¼ teaspoon freshly ground black pepper

1 small lemon

Fresh basil, or parsley, for garnish

Soy Parmesan cheese, for garnish (optional)

1. In a large glass baking dish, place the squash halves cut-side down. Add the water. Cover with plastic wrap. Microwave on high for 8 to 10 minutes, or until tender. Set aside.

2. While the squash cooks, place a large skillet over medium-high heat. Add 1½ teaspoons of olive oil.

3. Add the red onion. Cook for 3 minutes, or until translucent.

4. Add the zucchini. Cook for 4 to 5 minutes more, or until the zucchini browns.

5. Add the tomato, salt, oregano, basil, and pepper. Reduce the heat to low. Gently simmer for 10 minutes.

6. With a fork, scrape the cooked squash strands into a bowl. Add the remaining 1½ teaspoons of olive oil. Toss to coat.

7. Mound the squash onto a serving platter. Spoon the vegetable mixture around the squash. Drizzle with additional olive oil, if desired.

8. Squeeze the lemon over the vegetables. Garnish with the basil and soy Parmesan cheese (if using).

PER SERVING Calories: 195; Total Fat: 7g; Protein: 4g; Carbohydrates: 32g; Sugars: 14g; Fiber: 6g; Sodium: 359mg

TOSS IT TOGETHER TIP: *Leftover spaghetti squash can be frozen so that when a pasta craving strikes, all you have to do is defrost a bag. After cooking the squash, carefully remove as much excess water as you can by blotting and pressing the strands between paper towels. Freeze in small portions to maintain good texture.*

Porcini Mushroom Gravy

DAIRY-FREE
MAKES 2 CUPS • PREP TIME: 5 MINUTES • COOK TIME: 20 MINUTES

If you're looking for authentic mushroom flavor, dried porcini will not disappoint. Porcini mushrooms have a robust, earthy flavor and heady aroma that is fantastic for making truly amazing soups, sauces, and, in this recipe, a rich and delicious low-carb gravy. The mushrooms are reconstituted to their full meaty form to create a hearty gravy for your next Thanksgiving, or as a topping for grains, beans, or meats. To keep the carb count low, coconut flour is used for thickening.

½ cup dried porcini mushrooms

3¼ cups water, divided

2 tablespoons coconut flour

2 tablespoons extra-virgin olive oil

1 medium red onion, finely diced

2 garlic cloves, minced

1 teaspoon dried thyme

1 teaspoon dried rosemary

1 cup vegetable broth

½ teaspoon salt

Freshly ground black pepper, to season

1. In a medium bowl, combine the porcini mushrooms and 3 cups of water. Soak for 30 minutes.

2. In a small bowl, whisk the coconut flour and remaining ¼ cup of water into a thick paste. Set aside.

3. In a medium skillet set over medium-high heat, heat the olive oil.

4. Add the red onion. Cook for 3 minutes, or until browned.

5. Stir in the garlic, thyme, and rosemary. Cook for 1 minute.

6. Pour the porcini mushrooms, including their soaking water, into the skillet. Add the vegetable broth. Bring to a boil. Reduce the heat to low. Simmer for 15 minutes.

7. Place a fine mesh strainer over a large bowl. Pour the mushroom mixture into the strainer. Reserving the liquid in the bowl. Rinse the skillet. Put it back over medium-high heat.

8. Pour the reserved mushroom liquid into the skillet. Bring to a low boil.

(continued)

9. Add the coconut flour mixture. Stir well to combine. Continue to cook for 1 to 2 minutes more, stirring, until the gravy begins to thicken.

10. Add the strained mushrooms to the skillet. Add salt. Season with pepper. Cook, stirring, for 1 minute more.

11. Serve over quinoa, potatoes, or pasta, or use as a side dish.

PER SERVING (¼ cup) Calories: 95; Total Fat: 4g; Protein: 5g; Carbohydrates: 10g; Sugars: 2g; Fiber: 4g; Sodium: 163mg

INGREDIENT TIP: *Dried mushrooms may, at first, seem expensive but, when soaked in water, they rehydrate to 6 to 8 times their dry weight! They need no refrigeration, will keep many months in the pantry (longer in the freezer), and are ready at a moment's notice. Add to all of your favorite dishes for additional flavor.*

Tofu-Cilantro Sauce

QUICK & EASY

MAKES 2½ CUPS • PREP TIME: 5 MINUTES • COOK TIME: 5 MINUTES

Tofu is the perfect ingredient for casseroles, stir-fries, curries, lasagna, puddings, pies, and smoothies. It also makes an excellent base for sauces. High in protein with no saturated fat, cholesterol, or carbs, this plant-powered source of nutrition has a neutral taste that takes on the flavors of the herbs and spices used to season it. This delicious and creamy cilantro sauce works well over vegetables, pasta, grains, or beans.

1 pound firm tofu, drained, cut into 8 pieces

¼ cup plain nonfat Greek yogurt

1 teaspoon stone-ground mustard

3 tablespoons freshly squeezed lemon juice

1 tablespoon coarsely chopped fresh cilantro

1 garlic clove, minced

¼ teaspoon salt

¼ teaspoon paprika

1. Prepare a steamer.

2. In steamer basket, place the tofu. Steam for 3 to 5 minutes. Set aside.

3. In a blender, purée the yogurt, mustard, lemon juice, cilantro, garlic, salt, and paprika.

4. Add in 1 piece of tofu at a time and blend until smooth. Continue until all the tofu is blended in.

5. Serve warm.

PER SERVING (¼ cup) Calories: 39; Total Fat: 2g; Protein: 5g; Carbohydrates: 0g; Sugars: 0g; Fiber: 0g; Sodium: 65mg

INGREDIENT TIP: Firm tofu is a good choice when you want a sauce with a thicker consistency. Silken tofu is best suited for smoothies, puddings, and desserts. Extra-firm tofu is the best choice for stir-fries and for crumbling in place of cheese in lasagna.

Barbecue Sauce

DAIRY-FREE • QUICK & EASY
MAKES 1 CUP • PREP TIME: 5 MINUTES • COOK TIME: 5 MINUTES

If you have been searching for a low-carb, sugar-free barbecue sauce to use with your favorite recipes, look no further. This recipe uses plain tomato sauce and paste with a touch of mustard, paprika, and liquid smoke to give it characteristic barbecue flavors. Natural plant-based stevia is added for a hint of sweetness. Adjust the seasonings according to your taste preferences and enjoy this healthy alternative on all your favorite barbecued foods.

½ cup tomato sauce

2 tablespoons tomato paste

1 tablespoon balsamic vinegar

½ teaspoon dry mustard

1 garlic clove, minced

½ teaspoon smoked paprika

1 teaspoon liquid smoke

1 tablespoon granulated stevia

⅛ teaspoon salt

Freshly ground black pepper, to season

1. To a food processor or blender, add the tomato sauce, tomato paste, balsamic vinegar, dry mustard, garlic, smoked paprika, liquid smoke, stevia, and salt. Season with pepper. Blend for about 1 minute, or until smooth.

2. To a small saucepan set over medium-low heat, transfer the blended ingredients. Cover and bring to a light boil. Boil for 5 minutes. Remove from the heat.

3. Cool the sauce and refrigerate in an airtight container for up to 2 weeks.

PER SERVING (¼ cup) Calories: 42; Total Fat: 0g; Protein: 2g; Carbohydrates: 9g; Sugars: 5g; Fiber: 2g; Sodium: 393mg

INGREDIENT TIP: *Liquid smoke really is made from smoke. Chips or sawdust from hardwoods such as hickory or mesquite are burned at high temperatures, and particles of smoke are collected in condensers. The resulting liquid is concentrated for a stronger flavor. A little goes a long way, so experiment with quantities in recipes. Use liquid smoke to add a smoky flavor to meatloaf, fajitas, pulled pork, pasta, potatoes, and steak dishes.*

Fresh Cranberry Sauce

DAIRY-FREE • QUICK & EASY
MAKES 2 CUPS • PREP TIME: 1 MINUTE • COOK TIME: 5 MINUTES

Why eat cranberry sauce out of a can when you can whip up this nutritious and naturally sweetened sauce in a jiffy? Both fresh and frozen cranberries are available year-round at most supermarkets, and either works well in this recipe. The berries are simply boiled, processed gently, and sweetened with stevia to make this sauce. Full of antioxidants and vitamin C, this will boost the flavor of any dish. Serve as a side to grilled or baked fish, mix into oatmeal, add to pancakes, or proudly serve at your next holiday meal.

2 cups fresh cranberries, or frozen cranberries

1 tablespoon granulated stevia

¾ cup water

1. In a 4-quart saucepan set over medium heat, mix together the cranberries, stevia, and water. Cook for 1 minute, stirring constantly until the stevia dissolves. Bring to a boil. Cook for about 5 minutes more, or until the skins burst.

2. To a food processor or blender, transfer the cooked cranberries. Pulse gently for about 30 seconds.

3. Serve warm or chilled.

PER SERVING (½ cup) Calories: 15; Total Fat: 0g; Protein: 0g; Carbohydrates: 3g; Sugars: 1g; Fiber: 1g; Sodium: 0mg

TOSS IT TOGETHER TIP: *Add this sauce to smoothies, use as a relish for a baked sweet potato, add to tuna salad, barbecue sauce, or a stuffing for baked acorn squash. It is also a delicious replacement for high-sugar jam on toast, atop a burger, or frozen in small portions so you always have some on hand. The possibilities are limitless!*

Teriyaki Sauce

DAIRY-FREE • QUICK & EASY
MAKES 1 CUP • PREP TIME: 5 MINUTES • COOK TIME: 15 MINUTES

"Teriyaki" has become a catch-all term for various soy-based sweet-and-salty Asian sauces. Heavily flavored, teriyaki sauce usually contains ginger, garlic, sugar, and sesame seeds. When you make your own using only a handful of ingredients, you can eliminate excess sugar, carbs, and calories, but still have authentic flavors. Use this sauce in place of bottled teriyaki sauce to season all of your favorite Asian dishes.

½ cup low-sodium soy sauce

½ cup water

¼ cup granulated stevia

1 tablespoon ginger purée

1 tablespoon finely minced fresh garlic

1. In a small saucepan set over medium-high heat, stir together the soy sauce, water, stevia, ginger, and garlic. Simmer for about 15 minutes, or until reduced by about one-third to one-half.

2. Refrigerate until needed.

PER SERVING (2 tablespoons) Calories: 13; Total Fat: 0g; Protein: 1g; Carbohydrates: 2g; Sugars: 0g; Fiber: 0g; Sodium: 575mg

Easy Ketchup

DAIRY-FREE • QUICK & EASY
MAKES 1½ CUPS • PREP TIME: 5 MINUTES

Condiments add a kick to many dishes, and these jars of flavor have become essential to cooking and eating many favorite foods. But sometimes those additions aren't doing your health any favors. Bottled ketchup, while low fat, is high in sugar and sodium—especially if you are generous with the serving size. Skip the carbs and whip up this healthy homemade ketchup instead. Plain and simple tomato sauce serves as the base, and stevia sweetens it naturally. Authentic ketchup flavor is achieved with a combination of commonly available spices.

1 (6-ounce) can tomato paste

2 tablespoons apple cider vinegar

¼ teaspoon granulated stevia

¾ teaspoon salt

¾ teaspoon granulated garlic

¾ teaspoon granulated onion

¼ teaspoon ground allspice

⅔ cup water

1. In a bowl, mix together the tomato paste, apple cider vinegar, stevia, salt, garlic, onion, allspice, and water. Stir to blend completely.

2. Refrigerate until needed.

PER SERVING (2 tablespoons) Calories: 15; Total Fat: 0g; Protein: 1g; Carbohydrates: 3g; Sugars: 1g; Fiber: 0g; Sodium: 10mg

Spicy Peanut Sauce

DAIRY-FREE • QUICK & EASY
MAKES 2 CUPS • PREP TIME: 5 MINUTES • COOK TIME: 5 MINUTES

This delicious Asian-style peanut sauce uses stevia for a hint of sweetness and a dash of cayenne for just the right amount of kick. Serve with vegetables "noodles," over cooked grains, as a topping to sautéed beans, or with roasted vegetables. It also makes a nutritious dip for raw vegetables.

1 cup unsalted natural peanut butter (no sugar added)

1 cup water

1 tablespoon low-sodium soy sauce

1 tablespoon granulated stevia

¼ teaspoon salt

Dash cayenne pepper

¼ cup chopped scallions

Olive oil cooking spray

1. To a medium bowl, add the peanut butter. While whisking to blend, gradually add the water.

2. Whisk in the soy sauce, stevia, salt, cayenne pepper, and scallions.

3. Coat a saucepan with cooking spray.

4. Transfer the ingredients to the prepared pan. Cook for 5 minutes over low heat, stirring constantly, until heated through. The sauce will thicken as it warms.

5. Refrigerate any remaining sauce. Rewarm before using, if desired.

PER SERVING (2 tablespoons) Calories: 92; Total Fat: 7g; Protein: 4g; Carbohydrates: 3g; Sugars: 1g; Fiber: 1g; Sodium: 72mg

Chunky Red Pepper and Tomato Sauce

DAIRY-FREE

MAKES 2½ CUPS • PREP TIME: 5 MINUTES • COOK TIME: 40 MINUTES

While this recipe requires a bit of cooking time, the result is well worth it. Intense in flavor, this chunky red pepper and tomato sauce is made by roasting red peppers, sautéing them with a mix of aromatic herbs, and processing them with tomato purée. The result is a rich and hearty sauce that is also full of good-for-your-health vitamins, minerals, and antioxidants. This delicious sauce works well on grains, vegetables, potatoes, pasta, and other dishes.

3 large red bell peppers, halved lengthwise, seeded, pressed open to flatten

2 tablespoons extra-virgin olive oil, plus additional for brushing the peppers

1 medium onion, minced

1½ teaspoons dried basil

1 teaspoon dried rosemary

½ teaspoon dried oregano

½ teaspoon salt

½ cup low-sodium vegetable broth

2 cups water

½ cup tomato purée

1 tablespoon tomato paste

2 teaspoons white wine vinegar

2 tablespoons chopped fresh basil leaves

1. Preheat the broiler to high.

2. Brush the red bell peppers with olive oil. Place them under the broiler, skin-side up. Cook for about 10 minutes, or until lightly charred. Transfer the peppers to a cutting board, stacking one on top of the other to create steam. Let sit for 10 minutes. Remove as much charred skin as possible. Slice into strips.

3. In a large skillet set over medium-high heat, heat the remaining 2 tablespoons of olive oil.

4. Add the red pepper strips, onion, basil, rosemary, oregano, and salt. Cook for 5 minutes, stirring.

5. Add the vegetable broth. Cook for about 15 minutes more, or until the mixture reduces to a sauce.

6. Add the water, tomato purée, and tomato paste. Reduce the heat to low. Simmer for 25 minutes.

7. Transfer the mixture to a food processor. Purée until smooth, but with some texture remaining.

8. Place the skillet back over low heat. Return the sauce to the skillet. Barely simmer for 1 to 2 minutes to rewarm. Stir in the white wine vinegar and basil. Serve warm.

9. Refrigerate any remaining sauce. Serve chilled or rewarmed, as desired.

PER SERVING (¼ cup) Calories: 43; Total Fat: 3g; Protein: 0g; Carbohydrates: 4g; Sugars: 2g; Fiber: 1g; Sodium: 127mg

"Honey" Mustard Sauce

QUICK & EASY

MAKES ½ CUP • PREP TIME: 5 MINUTES

This recipe gives sugar- and carb-filled honey mustard sauce a nutritional makeover. High-protein Greek yogurt is mixed with tangy cider vinegar, a dash of dry mustard, smoky paprika, and naturally sweetened with stevia. Quick to assemble, make this homemade condiment for a smart food swap that will boost the quality of your diet. Use on baked chicken wings, chicken tenders, potatoes, in salads, and as a dipping sauce. Adjust the seasonings to suit your preferences.

½ cup plain nonfat
   Greek yogurt
1 tablespoon apple
   cider vinegar
1 teaspoon dry mustard
¾ teaspoon garlic powder
⅛ teaspoon paprika
1 tablespoon granulated stevia

1. In a small bowl, whisk together the yogurt, apple cider vinegar, dry mustard, garlic powder, paprika, and stevia until smooth.

2. Refrigerate until needed.

PER SERVING (2 tablespoons) Calories: 18; Total Fat: 0g; Protein: 3g; Carbohydrates: 1g; Sugars: 1g; Fiber: 0g; Sodium: 12mg

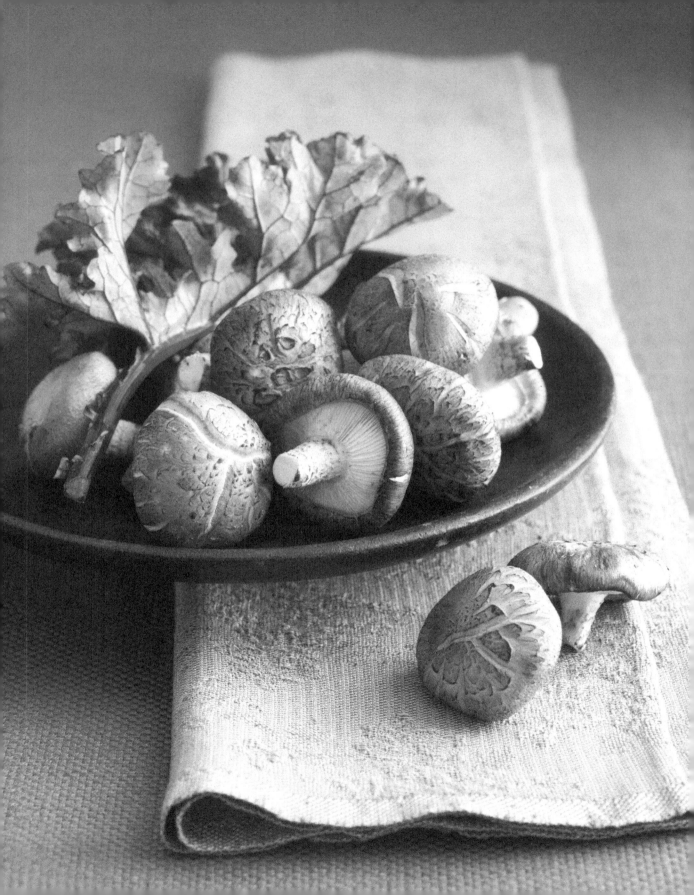

APPENDIX A

DIRTY DOZEN and CLEAN FIFTEEN

A nonprofit and environmental watchdog organization called Environmental Working Group (EWG) looks at data supplied by the U.S. Department of Agriculture (USDA) and the Food and Drug Administration (FDA) about pesticide residues and compiles a list each year of the best and worst pesticide loads found in commercial crops. You can use these lists to decide which fruits and vegetables to buy organic to minimize your exposure to pesticides and which produce is considered safe enough to skip the organics. This does not mean they are pesticide-free, though, so wash these fruits and vegetables thoroughly.

These lists change every year, so make sure you look up the most recent before you fill your shopping cart. You'll find the most recent lists as well as a guide to pesticides in produce at http://EWG.org/FoodNews.

The 2015 DIRTY DOZEN

- Apples
- Celery
- Cherry tomatoes
- Cucumbers
- Grapes
- Nectarines
- Peaches
- Potatoes
- Snap peas
- Spinach
- Strawberries
- Sweet bell peppers

Plus produce contaminated with highly toxic organophosphate insecticides:

- Hot peppers
- Kale/Collard greens

The CLEAN 15

- Asparagus
- Avocados
- Cabbage
- Cantaloupe
- Cauliflower
- Eggplant
- Grapefruit
- Kiwi
- Mangos
- Onions
- Papayas
- Pineapples
- Sweet corn
- Sweet peas (frozen)
- Sweet potatoes

CONVERSION TABLES

VOLUME EQUIVALENTS (LIQUID)

U.S. STANDARD	U.S. STANDARD (OUNCES)	METRIC (APPROXIMATE)
2 tablespoons	1 fl. oz.	30 mL
¼ cup	2 fl. oz.	60 mL
½ cup	4 fl. oz.	120 mL
1 cup	8 fl. oz.	240 mL
1½ cups	12 fl. oz.	355 mL
2 cups or 1 pint	16 fl. oz.	475 mL
4 cups or 1 quart	32 fl. oz.	1 L
1 gallon	128 fl. oz.	4 L

OVEN TEMPERATURES

FAHRENHEIT (F)	CELSIUS (C) (APPROXIMATE)
250	120
300	150
325	165
350	180
375	190
400	200
425	220
450	230

VOLUME EQUIVALENTS (DRY)

U.S. STANDARD	METRIC (APPROXIMATE)
⅛ teaspoon	0.5 mL
¼ teaspoon	1 mL
½ teaspoon	2 mL
¾ teaspoon	4 mL
1 teaspoon	5 mL
1 tablespoon	15 mL
¼ cup	59 mL
⅓ cup	79 mL
½ cup	118 mL
⅔ cup	156 mL
¾ cup	177 mL
1 cup	235 mL
2 cups or 1 pint	475 mL
3 cups	700 mL
4 cups or 1 quart	1 L
½ gallon	2 L
1 gallon	4 L

WEIGHT EQUIVALENTS

U.S. STANDARD	METRIC (APPROXIMATE)
½ ounce	15 g
1 ounce	30 g
2 ounces	60 g
4 ounces	115 g
8 ounces	225 g
12 ounces	340 g
16 ounces or 1 pound	455 g

GLOSSARY

antioxidant: A substance such as vitamin E, vitamin C, or beta-carotene, thought to protect the body's cells from the damaging effects of oxidation.

carbohydrate (simple and complex): Carbohydrates are divided into two groups: simple and complex, based on their chemical structure and how quickly sugar is digested and absorbed.

Simple carbohydrates are chemically made of one or two sugars and include sugars like soda and candy, but also nutrient-rich foods like fruit and milk. They are absorbed quickly into the bloodstream.

Complex carbohydrates are also known as starches and are made of three or more linked sugars. They include oatmeal, rice, pasta, and other grains, as well as some vegetables like broccoli and corn, and legumes and beans. They are digested slowly.

diabetes (type 1 and type 2): *Type 1 diabetes* is an autoimmune disease of the insulin-producing cells of the pancreas. It cannot be prevented and requires insulin injections. In *type 2 diabetes*, the body cannot use insulin properly. As the disease progresses, the pancreas makes less insulin, necessitating treatment with medications. Most type 2 diabetes cases can be prevented by maintaining a healthy weight and exercising.

FIFO: First in, first out. A system of labeling foods with the dates you get them or want to use them by and putting the older foods in front, or on top, so you use them first.

food exchanges: Exchanges are foods grouped together into categories or lists, according to their similarities in nutritional values. Measured portions of foods within each category may be exchanged for each other when planning meals. A single exchange contains about an equal amount of carbohydrates, protein, fat, and calories.

insulin: A hormone produced in the pancreas that regulates the amount of glucose (sugar) in the blood.

isoflavone: A phytoestrogen chiefly produced by plants of the legume family, especially soybeans, potentially useful in lowering cholesterol.

LDL cholesterol: A blood-plasma lipoprotein that is high in cholesterol and low in protein content and that carries cholesterol to cells and tissues; also called bad cholesterol.

marinate: To soak meat, fish, or vegetables in a sauce to tenderize and enrich the flavor.

phytochemical/phytonutrient: A nonnutritive bioactive plant substance, such as a flavonoid or carotenoid, considered to have a beneficial effect on human health.

ramekin: A small ceramic bowl for baking and serving.

whole grains: Whole grains contain all three parts of the wheat kernel: bran, germ, and endosperm. In contrast, refined grains only retain the endosperm.

RESOURCES

About.com home cooking. http://homecooking.about.com

American Diabetes Association. www.diabetes.org

Allrecipes. *Diabetic Recipes.* http://allrecipes.com/recipes/everyday-cooking/special-diets /diabetic/

Bragg Liquid Aminos. http://bragg.com/products/bragg-liquid-aminos-soy-alternative.html

Diabetes Health Center. http://www.webmd.com/diabetes/default.htm

Diabetes Information Hub. http://diabetesinformationhub.com

Diabetes Low-Carb Resources. http://diabetes-low-carb.org

Diabetes Research Institute. http://www.diabetesresearch.org/diabetes-research-institute

Eating Well's Recipes for Two. http://www.eatingwell.com/recipes_menus/recipes_for_two

Food Network's Diabetic Recipes. http://www.foodnetwork.com/topics/diabetes-friendly. html?vty=topics/diabetic.html

Ian's Panko Bread Crumbs. iansnaturalfoods.com/product-category/culinary-creations/

Joslin Diabetes Center: Diabetes Research, Care, Education, & Resources. http://www.joslin.org

Low-Carb Diabetic Recipes. http://www.easy-diabetic-recipes.com/low-carb-diabetic-recipes.html

Menu Planning for Your Diabetes Life. http://www.dlife.com/diabetes-food-and-fitness /what_do_i_eat/meal_planning

University of California, San Francisco. Diabetes Education Online. http://dtc.ucsf.edu

World's Healthiest Foods. http://www.whfoods.com

REFERENCES

ADA (American Diabetes Association). *The Official Pocket Guide to Diabetic Exchanges: Choose Your Foods.* Alexandria, VA: ADA, 2011.

Bernstein, Richard K. *The Diabetes Diet: Dr. Bernstein's Low-Carbohydrate Solution.* New York: Little, Brown and Company, 2005.

Bernstein, Richard K. *Dr. Bernstein's Diabetes Solution: The Complete Guide to Achieving Normal Blood Sugars.* 4th ed. New York: Little, Brown and Company, 2011.

Diabetic Living, eds. *Diabetes Meals by the Plate: 90 Low-Carb Meals to Mix & Match.* Des Moines, IA: Meredith Corp., 2014.

Elliot, Rose. *The Vegetarian Low-Carb Diet: The Fast, No-Hunger Weight Loss Diet for Vegetarians.* London: Piatkus Books, 2006.

"Healthy Eating: Easy Tips for Planning a Healthy Diet and Sticking to It." http://www.helpguide.org/articles/healthy-eating/healthy-eating.htm#tip1.

Hughes, Nancy. *Diabetes Carb Control Cookbook: Over 150 Recipes with Exactly 15 Grams of Carb—Perfect for Carb Counters!* Alexandria, VA: American Diabetes Association, 2014.

LaRue, Jacqueline. *The CarbLow Diet Diabetic Friendly 2015 Incredibly Quick Weight Loss via Carb Counting With CarbLow Cookbook.* Cookbooks from Around the World Publishers, 2014. Nook edition.

Mayo Clinic. *Mayo Clinic Essential Book of Diabetes: How to Prevent, Control, and Live Well with Diabetes.* 2nd ed. Birmingham, AL: Oxmoor House, 2014.

Phinney, Stephen, and Jeff Volek. *The Art and Science of Low Carbohydrate Living: An Expert Guide to Making the Life-Saving Benefits of Carbohydrate Restriction Sustainable and Enjoyable.* 1st ed. Miami: Beyond Obesity, 2011.

Porter, Jen. *Diabetes Diet Cookbook: Delicious Low Carb Recipes for Diabetics (Diabetes Miracle Cure, Lower Blood Sugar, Diabetes Desserts).* Amazon Digital Services, 2014. Kindle edition.

Richards, Oliver. *Tasty Diabetic Breakfast Recipes: For Low-Carb Eaters and Diabetics.* Amazon Digital Services, 2014. Kindle edition.

Webb, Robyn. *The American Diabetes Association Diabetes Comfort Food Cookbook.* Alexandria, VA: American Diabetes Association, 2011.

RECIPE INDEX

INDEX

CPSIA information can be obtained
at www.ICGtesting.com
Printed in the USA
BVOW05s1840070617
486310BV00011B/35/P